It's easy to get lost in the cancer world

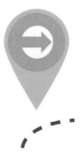

Let NCCN Guidelines for Patients® be your guide

✓ Step-by-step guides to the cancer care options likely to have the best results

✓ Based on treatment guidelines used by health care providers worldwide

✓ Designed to help you discuss cancer treatment with your doctors

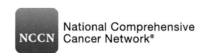

National Comprehensive Cancer Network®

NCCN Guidelines for Patients® are developed by the National Comprehensive Cancer Network® (NCCN®)

NCCN®

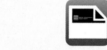

NCCN Clinical Practice Guidelines in Oncology (NCCN Guidelines®)

NCCN Guidelines for Patients®

✓ An alliance of leading cancer centers across the United States devoted to patient care, research, and education

Cancer centers that are part of NCCN:
NCCN.org/cancercenters

✓ Developed by doctors from NCCN cancer centers using the latest research and years of experience

✓ For providers of cancer care all over the world

✓ Expert recommendations for cancer screening, diagnosis, and treatment

Free online at
NCCN.org/guidelines

✓ Present information from the NCCN Guidelines in an easy-to-learn format

✓ For people with cancer and those who support them

✓ Explain the cancer care options likely to have the best results

Free online at
NCCN.org/patientguidelines

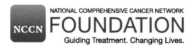

NATIONAL COMPREHENSIVE CANCER NETWORK
FOUNDATION
Guiding Treatment. Changing Lives.

and supported by funding from NCCN Foundation®

These NCCN Guidelines for Patients® are based on the NCCN Clinical Practice Guidelines in Oncology (NCCN Guidelines®) for Breast Cancer (Version 3.2020, March 6, 2020).

NCCN Foundation® seeks to support the millions of patients and their families affected by a cancer diagnosis by funding and distributing NCCN Guidelines for Patients®. NCCN Foundation is also committed to advancing cancer treatment by funding the nation's promising doctors at the center of innovation in cancer research. For more details and the full library of patient and caregiver resources, visit NCCN.org/patients.

National Comprehensive Cancer Network® (NCCN®) / NCCN Foundation®
3025 Chemical Road, Suite 100
Plymouth Meeting, PA 19462
215.690.0300

Endorsed by

Breast Cancer Alliance

Receiving a cancer diagnosis can be overwhelming, both for the patient and their family. We support the NCCN Guidelines for Patients: Invasive Breast Cancer with the knowledge that these tools will help to equip patients with many of the educational resources, and answers to questions, they may seek. breastcanceralliance.org

Breastcancer.org

Breastcancer.org is a leading resource for people to make sense of the complex medical and personal information about breast health and breast cancer. Our mission is to engage, educate, and empower people with expert information and our dynamic peer support community to help everyone make the best decisions for their lives. breastcancer.org

DiepCFoundation

DiepCFoundation applauds the National Comprehensive Cancer Network (NCCN) for their ongoing work in the development of Patient Guidelines. We endorse the NCCN Guidelines for Patients: Invasive Breast Cancer for patients seeking information about all options for breast reconstruction after cancer. The Principles of Breast Reconstruction Following Surgery in the NCCN Guidelines directly aligns with the mission of the Foundation to educate and empower more patients with the information needed to make an informed decision about breast reconstruction after surgical treatment for breast cancer. diepcfoundation.org

FORCE: Facing Our Risk of Cancer Empowered

As the nation's leading organization serving the hereditary cancer community, FORCE is pleased to endorse the NCCN Guidelines for Patients: Invasive Breast Cancer. This guide provides valuable, evidence-based, expert reviewed information on the standard of care, empowering patients to make informed decisions about their treatment. facingourrisk.org

Sharsheret

Sharsheret is proud to endorse this important resource, the NCCN Guidelines for Patients: Invasive Breast Cancer. With this critical tool in hand, women nationwide have the knowledge they need to partner with their healthcare team to navigate the often complicated world of breast cancer care and make informed treatment decisions. sharsheret.org

With generous support from

- Benjamin Anderson, MD, in honor of Joan McClure
- Patricia Andrews
- Kristina Griffin
- Kate Townsend

To make a gift or learn more, please visit NCCNFoundation.org/donate or e-mail PatientGuidelines@nccn.org.

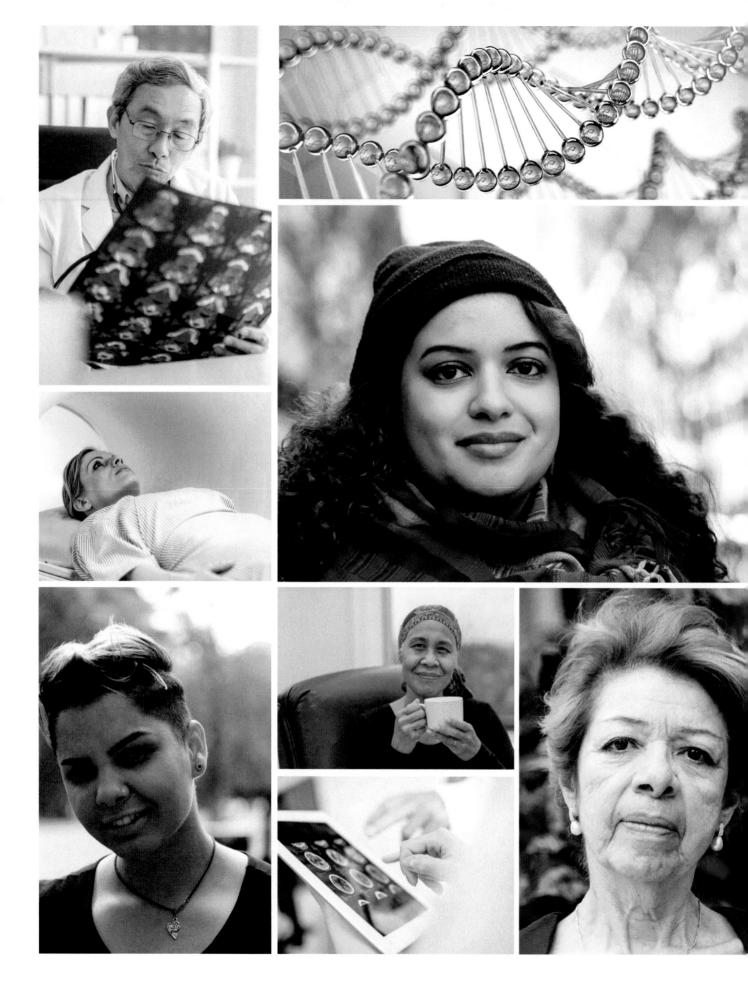

Contents

6   Breast cancer basics

14   Testing for breast cancer

28   Treatment options

41   Breast reconstruction

44   Stage 1, 2, and 3A

59   Stage 3

71   Recurrence

75   Inflammatory breast cancer

85   Making treatment decisions

94   Words to know

98   NCCN Contributors

99   NCCN Cancer Centers

100   Index

1
Breast cancer basics

7   The breast

8   Breast cancer

8   How breast cancer spreads

9   Cancer stages

11   Invasive breast cancer stages

13   Review

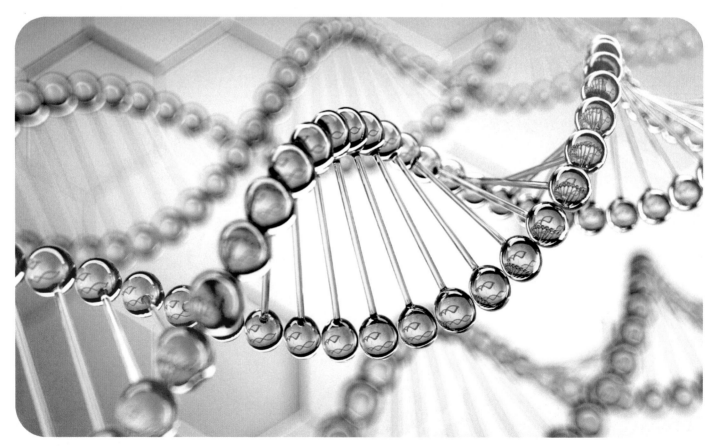

Breast cancer starts in the cells of the breast. Invasive breast cancer is cancer that has spread from the milk ducts or milk glands into the breast tissue or nearby lymph nodes.

The breast

The breast is an organ and a gland found on the chest. The breast is made of milk ducts, fat, nerves, lymph and blood vessels, ligaments, and other connective tissue. Behind the breast is the pectoral muscle and ribs. Muscle and ligaments help hold the breast in place.

Breast tissue contains glands that can make milk. These milk glands are called lobules. Lobules look like tiny clusters of grapes. Small tubes called ducts connect the lobules to the nipple.

The ring of darker breast skin is called the areola. The raised tip within the areola is called the nipple. The nipple-areola complex is a term that refers to both parts.

Lymph is a clear fluid that gives cells water and food. It also helps to fight germs. Lymph drains from breast tissue into lymph vessels and travels to lymph nodes near your armpit (axilla). Nodes near the armpit are called axillary lymph nodes (ALNs).

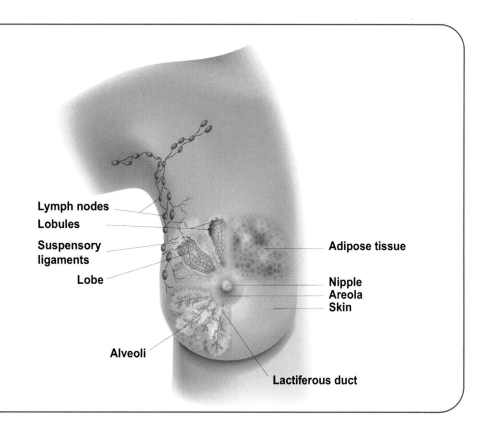

The breast

The breast is a glandular organ made up of milk ducts, fat, nerves, blood and lymph vessels, ligaments, and other connective tissue.

Lymph nodes
Lobules
Suspensory ligaments
Lobe
Adipose tissue
Nipple
Areola
Skin
Alveoli
Lactiferous duct

Breast cancer

Breast cancer starts in the cells of the breast. Almost all breast cancers are carcinomas. Carcinomas are cancers that start in the cells that line the inner or outer surfaces of the body.

There is more than one type of breast carcinoma.

> Ductal breast cancer starts in the cells that line the milk ducts. Milk ducts are thin tubes that carry milk from the lobules of the breast to the nipple. It is the most common type of breast cancer.

> Lobular breast cancer starts in the lobules (milk glands) of the breast.

Anyone can have breast cancer, including men. Although there are some differences between men and women, treatment is very similar.

How breast cancer spreads

Cancer cells don't behave like normal cells. Cancer cells differ from normal cells in the following ways.

Primary tumor
Over time, cancer cells form a mass called a primary tumor.

Invasive
Cancer cells can grow into surrounding tissues. Invasive breast cancer is breast cancer that has spread from the milk ducts or lobules into the breast tissue or nearby lymph nodes.

Metastasis
Unlike normal cells, cancer cells can spread and form tumors in other parts of the body. Cancer that has spread is called a metastasis. In this process, cancer cells break away from the first (primary) tumor and travel through blood or lymph vessels to distant sites. Once in other sites, cancer cells may form secondary tumors.

> Cancer that has spread to a nearby body part such as the axillary lymph nodes is called a local metastasis. It might be referred to as local/regional disease or locally advanced.

> Cancer that has spread to a body part far from the primary tumor is called a distant metastasis.

Breast cancer can metastasize to the bones, lungs, liver, spine, or brain. Breast cancer that has metastasized to other parts of the body is still called breast cancer.

Cancer stages

A cancer stage is a rating of the cancer based on test results. The American Joint Committee on Cancer (AJCC) created this to determine how much cancer is in your body, where it is located, and what subtype you have. This is called staging. Based on testing, your cancer will be assigned a stage. Staging is needed to make treatment decisions.

Cancer staging is often done twice.

> **Clinical stage (c)** is the rating given before any treatment. It is based on a physical exam, biopsy, and imaging tests. An example might look like cN2 or cM1.

> **Pathologic stage (p)** or surgical stage is determined by examining tissue removed during an operation. An example might be pN2. If you are given drug therapy before surgery, then the stage might look like ypT3.

Information gathered during staging:

> **The extent (size) of the tumor (T):** How large is the cancer? Has it grown into nearby areas?

> **The spread to nearby lymph nodes (N):** Has the cancer spread to nearby lymph nodes? If so, how many? Where?

> **The spread (metastasis) to distant sites (M):** Has the cancer spread to distant organs such as the lungs or liver?

> **Estrogen receptor (ER) status:** Does the cancer have the protein called an estrogen receptor?

> **Progesterone receptor (PR) status:** Does the cancer have the protein called a progesterone receptor?

> **Human epidermal growth factor receptor 2 (HER2) status:** Does the cancer make too much of a protein called HER2?

> **Grade of the cancer (G):** How much do the cancer cells look like normal cells?

TNM scores

The tumor, node, metastasis (TNM) system is used to stage breast cancer. In this system, the letters T, N, and M describe different areas of cancer growth. Based on cancer test results, your doctor will assign a score or number to each letter. The higher the number, the larger the tumor or the more the cancer has spread. These scores will be combined to assign the cancer a stage. A TNM example might look like this: T1N0M0 or T1, N0, M0.

> **T (tumor)** - Size of the main (primary) tumor

> **N (node)** - If cancer has spread to nearby (regional) lymph nodes

> **M (metastasis)** - If cancer has spread to distant parts of the body or metastasized

Numbered stages

Number stages range from stage 1 to stage 4, with 4 being the most advanced. Doctors write these stages as stage I, stage II, stage III, and stage IV.

Stage 0 is noninvasive

Noninvasive breast cancer is rated stage 0. This cancer is found only inside the ducts or lobules. It has not spread to surrounding breast tissue, lymph nodes (N0), or distant sites (M0).

Stages 1, 2, and 3 are invasive

Invasive breast cancer is rated stage 1, 2, or 3. It has grown outside the ducts, lobules, or breast skin. Cancer might be in the axillary lymph nodes.

Stage 4 is metastatic

In stage 4 breast cancer, cancer has spread to distant sites, but can also be found in the axillary lymph nodes. Your first diagnosis can be stage 4 metastatic breast cancer or it can develop from earlier stages.

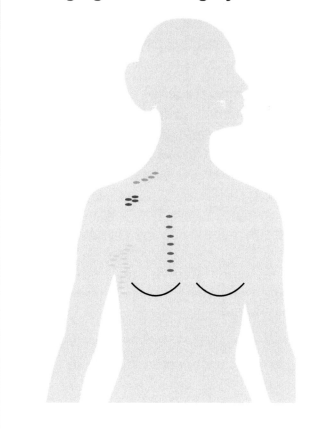

Clinical staging of lymph nodes is staging before surgery

Cancer is in **axillary nodes**

Cancer is in **internal mammary nodes**

Cancer is in infraclavicular nodes

Cancer is in supraclavicular nodes

Invasive breast cancer stages

Staging of invasive breast cancer is complex. It takes into account what can be felt during a physical exam, what can be seen on imaging tests, and what is found during a biopsy or surgery. Keep copies of your pathology reports. The pathology report might include a lot of abbreviations such as pN0(mol+), ypT2, or cN3. Your doctor can help explain what they mean.

The following section describes clinical staging of invasive breast cancer. These stages can be found in Guide 1.

Guide 1 — Invasive breast cancer stages		
Stage 1	**Stage 1A**	• T1, N0, M0
	Stage 1B	• T0, N1mi, M0 • T1, N1mi, M0
Stage 2	**Stage 2A**	• T0, N1, M0 • T1, N1, M0 • T2, N0, M0
	Stage 2B	• T2, N1, M0 • T3, N0, M0
Stage 3	**Stage 3A**	• T0, N2, M0 • T1, N2, M0 • T2, N2, M0 • T3, N1, M0 • T3, N2, M0
	Stage 3B	• T4, N0, M0 • T4, N1, M0 • T4, N2, M0
	Stage 3C	• Any T, N3, M0

T = Tumor

The primary tumor size can be measured in centimeters (cm) or millimeters (mm). A large pea is 1 cm (10 mm). A golf ball is 4 cm (40 mm). A micrometastasis is a very small cancerous cell that is smaller than 2 mm. It might be written as T1mi.

> **T1** Tumor is 2 cm or less

> **T1mi** Tumor is micrometastasis of 2 mm or less

> **T2** Tumor is 2.1 cm to 5 cm

> **T3** Tumor is more than 5 cm

> **T4** Tumor is of any size and has invaded nearby structures such the chest wall and skin of the breast

> **T4d** Inflammatory carcinoma

N = Node

There are hundreds of lymph nodes throughout your body. They work as filters to help fight infection and remove harmful things from your body. Regional lymph nodes are those located near the tumor in the breast. If breast cancer spreads, it often goes first to nearby lymph nodes under the arm. It can also sometimes spread to lymph nodes near the collarbone or near the breast bone. Knowing if the cancer has spread to your lymph nodes helps doctors find the best way to treat your cancer.

> **N0** means no cancer is in the regional lymph nodes.

> **N1, N2, N3** means regional lymph node metastases are found. The higher the number, the more lymph nodes that have metastases.

> **N1mi** means micrometastases are found in lymph nodes.

M = Metastatic

Cancer that has spread to distant parts of the body is shown as M1. The most common sites for metastasis are bone and lung.

> **M0** means no distant metastasis.

> **M1** means distant metastasis is found. This is metastatic breast cancer.

Review

> Inside breasts are lobules, milk ducts, fat, blood and lymph vessels, ligaments, and connective tissue. Lobules are structures that make breast milk. Ducts carry breast milk from the lobules to the nipple.

> Breast cancer often starts in the ducts or lobules and then spreads into the surrounding tissue.

> Breast cancer that is found only in the ducts or lobules is called noninvasive.

> Invasive breast cancer is cancer that has grown outside the ducts or lobules into surrounding tissue. Once outside the ducts or lobules, breast cancer can spread through lymph or blood to lymph nodes or other parts of the body.

> Metastatic breast cancer has spread to distant sites in the body.

> Anyone can have breast cancer, including men. Although there are some differences between men and women, treatment is very similar.

Pathology report

All lab results are included in a pathology report. This report is sent to your doctor who will share the results with you. Ask for a copy of the report.

2
Testing for breast cancer

15 General health tests

16 Fertility and birth control

17 Blood tests

17 Imaging

19 Tissue tests

22 Hormone receptor tests

23 Tumor tests

24 Genetic tests

25 Distress screening

26 Test results

27 Review

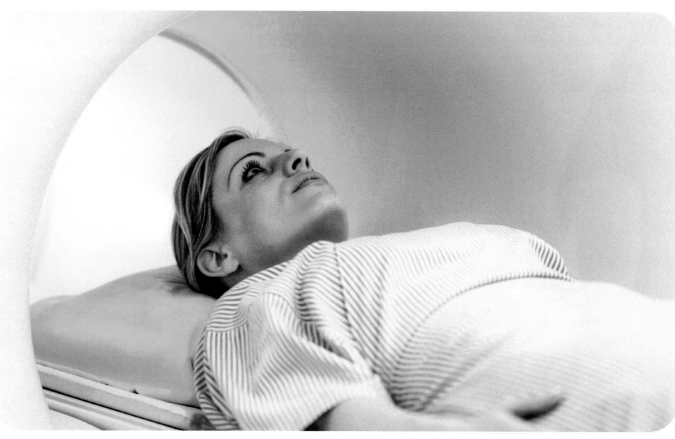

Not all invasive breast cancers are the same. Treatment planning starts with testing. This chapter presents an overview of the tests you might receive and what to expect.

General health tests

Medical history
A medical history is a record of all health issues and treatments you have had in your life. Be prepared to list any illness or injury and when it happened. Bring a list of old and new medicines and any over-the-counter medicines, herbs, or supplements you take. Tell your doctor about any symptoms you have. A medical history will help determine which treatment is best for you.

Family history
Some cancers and other diseases can run in families. Your doctor will ask about the health history of family members who are blood relatives. This information is called a family history. You can ask family members about their health issues like heart disease, cancer, and diabetes, and at what age they were diagnosed.

Physical exam
A physical exam is a study of your body. A doctor will check your body for signs of disease.

A health care provider may:

> Check your temperature, blood pressure, pulse, and breathing rate

> Weigh you

> Listen to your lungs and heart

> Look in your eyes, ears, nose, and throat

> Feel and apply pressure to parts of your body to see if organs are of normal size, are soft or hard, or cause pain when touched. Tell your doctor if you feel pain.

> Feel for enlarged lymph nodes in your neck and underarm. Tell the doctor if you have felt any lumps or have any pain.

> Complete a breast exam

Doctors should perform a thorough physical exam along with a complete health history.

Bring a list of any medications, vitamins, over-the-counter drugs, herbs, or supplements you are taking.

Fertility and birth control

Treatment can affect your fertility or your ability to have children. If you think you want children in the future, ask your doctor how cancer and cancer treatment will change your fertility and sexual health.

In order to preserve your fertility, you may need to take action before starting cancer treatment. Those who want to have children in the future should be referred to a fertility specialist before starting treatment to discuss the options.

More information can be found in NCCN *Guidelines for Patients®: Adolescents and Young Adults with Cancer*, available at NCCN.org/patientguidelines.

Those with ovaries

Those who can have children will have a pregnancy test before starting treatment. Cancer treatment can hurt the baby if you are or become pregnant during treatment. Therefore, birth control to prevent pregnancy during and after treatment is recommended. Hormonal birth control may not be recommended, so ask your doctor about options.

Those with testicles

Cancer and cancer treatment can damage sperm. Therefore, use contraception (birth control) to prevent pregnancy during and after cancer treatment. If you think you want children in the future, talk to your doctor now. Sperm banking is an option.

Infertility

Infertility is the complete loss of the ability to have children. The actual risk of infertility is related to your age at time of diagnosis, treatment type(s), treatment dose, and treatment length. Chemotherapy with alkylating agents has a higher risk of infertility. Sometimes, there isn't time for fertility preservation before you start treatment. Talk to your doctor about your concerns.

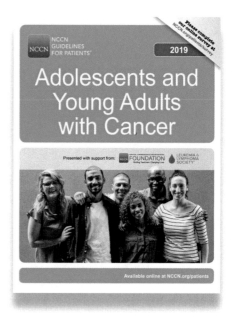

Blood tests

Blood tests check for signs of disease and how well organs are working. They require a sample of your blood, which is removed through a needle placed into your vein.

Pregnancy test

Those who can become pregnant will be given a pregnancy test before treatment begins.

Complete blood count

A complete blood count (CBC) measures the levels of red blood cells, white blood cells, and platelets in your blood. Your doctor will want to know if you have enough red blood cells to carry oxygen throughout your body, white blood cells to fight infection, and platelets to control bleeding.

Comprehensive metabolic panel

A comprehensive metabolic panel (CMP) is a test that measures 14 different substances in your blood. A CMP provides important information about how well your kidneys and liver are working, among other things. Creatinine is often part of a CMP. This test measures the health of your kidneys.

Liver function tests

Liver function tests (LFTs) look at the health of your liver by measuring chemicals that are made or processed by the liver. Levels that are too high or low signal that the liver is not working well.

Imaging

Imaging tests take pictures of the inside of your body. These tests are used to find and treat breast cancer. Imaging tests show the primary tumor, or where the cancer started, and look for cancer in other parts of the body.

A radiologist, an expert who looks at test images, will write a report and send this report to your doctor. Your doctor will discuss the results with you. Feel free to ask as many questions as you like.

Diagnostic mammogram

A mammogram is a picture of the insides of your breast. The pictures are made using x-rays. A computer combines the x-rays to make detailed pictures.

Diagnostic mammograms look at specific areas of your breast, which may not be clearly seen on screening mammograms. A bilateral mammogram includes pictures of both breasts. It is used to see if there is more than one tumor and the size of the tumor(s). Mammogram results are used to plan treatment. Other tests on your breast may be an ultrasound or breast MRI.

CT scan

A computed tomography (CT or CAT) scan uses x-rays and computer technology to take pictures of the inside of the body. It takes many x-rays of the same body part from different angles. All the images are combined to make one detailed picture.

A CT scan of your chest, abdomen, and/or pelvis may be one of the tests to look for cancer. In most cases, contrast will be used.

Contrast material is used to improve the pictures of the inside of the body. Contrast materials are not dyes, but substances that help certain areas in the body stand out. Contrast is used to make the pictures clearer.

Tell your doctors if you have had bad reactions to contrast in the past. This is important. You might be given medicines, such as Benadryl® and prednisone, for an allergy to contrast. Contrast might not be used if you have a serious allergy or if your kidneys aren't working well.

MRI scan

A magnetic resonance imaging (MRI) scan uses radio waves and powerful magnets to take pictures of the inside of the body. It does not use x-rays. Contrast might be used.

Breast MRI

If needed, a breast MRI would be used in addition to a mammogram. A breast MRI should be performed and interpreted by an expert breast imaging team working together with a multidisciplinary treatment team.

Spine and brain MRI

Breast cancer can spread (metastasize) to your spine or brain. Contrast should be used. For a brain MRI, a device is placed around your head that sends and receives radio waves. For spine MRI, no device is worn.

Bone scan

Breast cancer can spread to bones. A bone scan is an imaging test that can show if cancer has spread to your bones. This test may be used if you have bone pain, are at high risk for bone metastases, or if there are changes in certain test results. Bone scans might be used to monitor treatment. Your entire skeleton will be checked.

A bone scan uses a radiotracer to make pictures of the inside areas of your bone that are abnormal. A radiotracer is a substance that releases small amounts of radiation. Before the pictures are taken, the tracer will be injected into your vein. It can take a few hours for the tracer to enter your bones.

A special camera will take pictures of the tracer in your bones as it moves over your body. Areas of bone damage use more radiotracer than healthy bone and show up as bright spots on the pictures. Bone damage can be caused by cancer, cancer treatment, previous injuries, or other health problems.

Bone x-ray

An x-ray uses low-dose radiation to take one picture at a time. A tumor changes the way radiation is absorbed and will show up on the x-ray. X-rays are also good at showing bone problems. Your doctor may order x-rays if your bones hurt or were abnormal on a bone scan.

PET/CT scan

A positron emission tomography (PET) scan uses a radioactive drug called a tracer. A tracer is a substance put into your body to see how cancer is growing and where it is in the body. Cancer cells show up as bright spots on PET scans. Not all bright spots are cancer.

Sometimes CT is combined with PET. This combined test is called a PET/CT scan. It may be done with one or two machines depending on the cancer center.

Sodium fluoride PET/CT

A sodium fluoride PET/CT might be used instead of a bone scan. In this test, the radiotracer is made of sodium fluoride.

FDG PET/CT

An FDG PET/CT uses a radiotracer called F-18 fluorodeoxyglucose (FDG). It is made of fluoride and a simple form of sugar called glucose. You cannot eat or drink for at least 4 hours before the scan.

This scan is most helpful when other imaging results are unclear. It may help find cancer in lymph nodes and distant sites. If it clearly shows cancer in the bone, a bone scan and sodium fluoride PET/CT may not be needed. FDG PET/CT can be done at the same time as a CT used for diagnosis.

Ultrasound

An ultrasound uses high-energy sound waves to form pictures of the inside of the body. A probe will be held on your bare breast. It may also be placed below your armpit. Ultrasound is good at showing small areas of cancer that are near the surface of the body. Sometimes, an ultrasound or MRI is used to guide a biopsy.

Tissue tests

To confirm cancer is present, a tissue sample needs to be removed and tested. If cancer is confirmed, more lab tests will be done to learn about the cancer. Not all breast cancers are treated alike. Your doctor will use the lab results to decide which treatment options are right for you.

Biopsy

A biopsy is a procedure that removes a sample of tissue or fluid. The sample is sent to a lab for testing. A pathologist will test the biopsy for cancer and write a report called a pathology report. Ask questions about your biopsy results and what it means for your treatment.

There are different types of biopsies. Some biopsies are guided using imaging, such as an ultrasound or CT. The primary or main tumor is biopsied first. Other tumors or tumors in different areas may also be biopsied. You may have tissue removed from the breast, lymph nodes, or both.

Types of possible biopsies include:

> **Fine-needle aspiration (FNA)** uses a thin needle to remove a sample of tissue or fluid.

> **Core needle biopsy** removes tissue samples with a wide, hollow needle.

> **Incisional biopsy** removes a small amount of tissue through a cut in the skin or body.

A core needle biopsy removes more than one tissue sample. The samples are small. A "vacuum" may be used to remove a larger sample. The needle is often guided into the tumor with imaging. When mammography is used, it is called a stereotactic needle biopsy.

One or more clips may be placed near the breast tumor during a biopsy. The clips are small and made of metal. They will mark the site for future treatment and imaging. The clips stay in place and may be in your body for a period of time.

Sentinel lymph node biopsy

A sentinel lymph node is the first lymph node to which cancer cells are most likely to spread from a primary tumor. Sometimes, there can be more than one sentinel lymph node. A

sentinel lymph node biopsy (SLNB) is done during surgery such as a lumpectomy (surgery to remove a lump) or a mastectomy (surgery to remove the breast) to determine if any cancer cells have traveled to the lymph nodes. The removed lymph nodes are called sentinel lymph nodes. They may or may not contain any cancer cells. This biopsy is also called a sentinel node biopsy (SNB).

To find the sentinel lymph nodes, a radioactive material and other dyes are injected into the body near the breast where they travel through the lymphatics in the breast to the lymph nodes. This helps the surgeon find the sentinel lymph nodes. Once the nodes are found, one is removed and tested by a pathologist. If cancer is found, more than one lymph node may be removed.

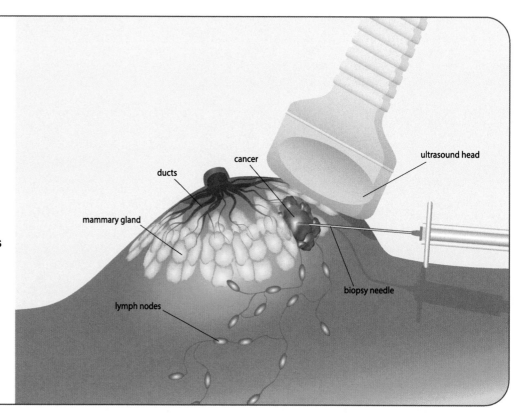

Biopsy

In a biopsy, a sample of tumor is removed. There are different types of biopsy. This image shows an ultrasound-guided needle biopsy.

ducts

cancer

ultrasound head

mammary gland

biopsy needle

lymph nodes

Axillary lymph node biopsy

An axillary lymph node (ALN) drains lymph from the breast and nearby areas. In an axillary lymph node biopsy, a sample of lymph node near the armpit (axilla) is biopsied with a needle. This is to determine if abnormal lymph nodes seen on imaging tests contain cancer cells. An ultrasound-guided fine-needle aspiration (US-FNA) or core biopsy will be used. If cancer is found, it is called node positive.

Axillary lymph node dissection

An axillary lymph node dissection (ALND) is surgery to remove axillary lymph nodes. This is performed after an ALN biopsy or SLNB shows cancer in the lymph nodes (called node positive). Then, an ALND will remove any other lymph nodes that contain cancer. Removing lymph nodes can cause lymphedema and other health issues.

There are 3 levels of axillary lymph nodes:

> **Level I** – nodes located below the lower edge of the chest muscle

> **Level II** – nodes located underneath the chest muscle

> **Level III** – nodes located above the chest muscle near the collarbone

An ALND usually removes level I and II axillary lymph nodes. For more information about the timing of biopsies, talk with your care team.

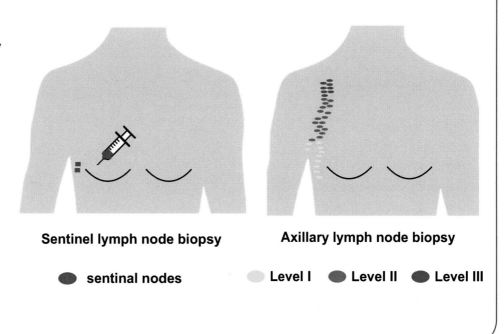

Lymph node surgery

There are two types of surgeries to remove lymph nodes. A sentinel lymph node biopsy finds and removes the lymph nodes where breast cancer first spreads. An axillary lymph node dissection removes lymph nodes from Levels I and II.

Sentinel lymph node biopsy

● sentinal nodes

Axillary lymph node biopsy

◯ Level I ● Level II ● Level III

Hormone receptor tests

A hormone is a substance made by a gland in your body. Your blood carries hormones throughout your body. A receptor is a protein found inside or on the surface of a cell. Substances such as hormones attach (bind) to these receptors. This causes changes within the cell.

Hormone receptors

Hormones recognize and bind to specific hormone receptors.

There are 2 types of hormone receptors:

> **Estrogen –** plays a role in breast development

> **Progesterone –** plays a role in menstrual cycle and pregnancy

Once these hormones attach to receptors inside breast cancer cells, they can cause cancer to grow. If found, these receptors may be targeted using endocrine therapy.

Immunohistochemistry

Immunohistochemistry (said immuno-histo-chemistry or IHC) is a special staining process that involves adding a chemical marker to cells. These cells are then studied using a microscope. IHC can find hormone receptors in breast cancer cells. A pathologist will measure how many cells have hormone receptors and the amount of hormone receptors inside each cell. Test results will either be hormone receptor-positive or hormone receptor-negative.

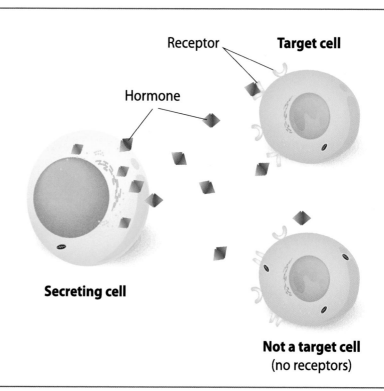

Hormone receptors

Cells in the ovaries, testes, and adrenal glands secrete hormones. Hormones recognize and bind to specific hormone receptors.

Receptor **Target cell**

Hormone

Secreting cell

Not a target cell (no receptors)

Hormone receptor-positive

In hormone receptor-positive (HR+) breast cancer, IHC finds estrogen and/or progesterone hormone receptors in at least 1 out of every 100 cancer cells. These cancers are sometimes simply called hormone positive. Most breast cancers are hormone positive.

There are 2 types of HR+ cells:

> Estrogen receptor-positive (ER+) cancer cells may need estrogen to grow. These cells may stop growing or die with treatment to block estrogen.

> Progesterone receptor-positive (PR+) cancer cells need progesterone to grow. These cells stop growing with treatment to block progesterone.

Hormone receptor-negative

Hormone receptor-negative (HR-) breast cancer cells do not have either estrogen or progesterone hormone receptors. These cancers are sometimes simply called hormone negative. Hormone-negative cancers often grow faster than hormone-positive cancers.

There are 2 types of HR- cells:

> Estrogen-receptor negative (ER-) cancer cells do not have an estrogen receptor. These cancer cells do not need estrogen to grow and continue to grow despite treatment to block estrogen.

> Progesterone-receptor negative (PR-) cancer cells do not need progesterone to grow. These cells continue to grow despite treatment to block progesterone.

Tumor tests

A sample from a biopsy of your tumor will be tested to look for biomarkers or proteins. This information is used to choose the best treatment for you. It is sometimes called molecular testing.

HER2

Human epidermal growth factor receptor 2 (HER2) is a protein found on the surface of breast cells. When amounts are high, it causes cells to grow and divide. Normal breast cells have two copies of the gene that makes HER2. They also have a normal number of HER2 on the cell surface.

In contrast to normal cells, some breast cancers have too many HER2 genes or receptors. Too many HER2s is called HER2-positive (HER2+).

There are 2 tests for HER2:

> **Immunohistochemistry (IHC)** measures receptors. If the IHC score is 3+, the cancer is HER2+.

> **In situ hybridization (ISH)** counts the number of copies of the *HER2* gene.

You might have more than one HER2 test. HER2 tests are done using a biopsy sample.

Tumor mutation testing

A sample of your tumor or blood may be used to see if the cancer cells have any specific mutations. Some mutations can be targeted with specific therapies. This is separate from the genetic testing for mutations that you may have inherited from your parents. An example of this is a mutation in a gene known as *PIK3CA*.

PD-L1 testing

Programmed death-ligand 1 (PD-L1) is an immune system protein. This protein can cause your immune cells to ignore the cancer cells and suppress the anti-tumor immune response. If any of the cells in your tumor sample have (express) the PD-L1 protein, you might have treatment that combines chemotherapy and immunotherapy. This is designed to activate your immune system to better fight off the cancer cells.

MSI/MMR testing

MSI

Microsatellites are short, repeated strings of DNA (the information inside genes). When errors or defects occur, they are fixed. Some cancers prevent these errors from being fixed. This is called microsatellite instability (MSI). Knowing this can help plan treatment.

MMR

Mismatch repair (MMR) helps fix mutations in certain genes. When MMR is lacking (dMMR), these mutations may lead to cancer. Knowing this can help plan treatment or predict how well treatment will work with your type of tumor. When cancer cells have more than a normal number of microsatellites, it is called MSI-H (microsatellite instability-high).

Other tumor testing

Your blood or biopsy may be tested for proteins. These proteins are called tumor markers. Knowing this information can help plan treatment. Examples of some tumor markers in breast cancer include carcinoembryonic antigen (CEA), CA 15-3, and CA 27.29. An increase in the level of certain tumor markers could mean that the cancer has grown or spread (progressed).

> Genetic testing is recommended for all men with breast cancer.

Genetic tests

Anything that increases your chances of cancer is called a risk factor. Risk factors can be activities that people do, things you have contact with in the environment, or traits passed down from parents to children through genes (inherited or hereditary). Genes are coded instructions that tell your cells what to do and what to become. An abnormal change in these instructions—called a gene mutation—can cause cells to grow and divide out of control.

Genetics can increase the risk of breast cancer. Your disease or family history may suggest you have hereditary breast cancer.

Your health care provider might refer you for genetic testing to learn more about your risk of developing breast cancer or other cancers. A genetic counselor will speak to you about the results. A genetic counselor is an expert who has special training in genetic diseases and will explain your chances of having hereditary breast cancer.

Genetic counseling

Your genetic counselor or oncologist might recommend genetic testing. *BRCA1* and *BRCA2* gene mutations are related to breast cancer. Other genes may be tested as well. Tests results may be used to guide treatment planning.

BRCA tests

Everyone has genes called *BRCA1* and *BRCA2*. Normal *BRCA* genes help to prevent tumor growth. They help fix damaged cells and help cells grow normally. *BRCA1* and *BRCA2* mutations put you as risk for more than one type of cancer. Mutations in *BRCA1* or *BRCA2* increase the risk of breast, ovarian, prostate, colorectal, or melanoma skin cancer. Mutated *BRCA* genes can also affect how well some treatments work. Your doctor might choose a treatment that is known to work better for your mutation.

Distress screening

Distress is an unpleasant experience of a mental, physical, social, or spiritual nature. It can affect how you feel, think, and act. Distress might include feelings of sadness, fear, helplessness, worry, anger, and guilt. You may also experience depression, anxiety, and sleeping problems.

It is normal to have strong feelings about being diagnosed with cancer. Talk to your doctor and with those whom you feel most comfortable about how you are feeling. There are services and people who can help you. Support and counseling are available.

Dealing with a cancer diagnosis is stressful and may cause distress. Your treatment team will screen your level of distress. This is part of your cancer care.

For more information, read the *NCCN Guidelines for Patients®: Distress*, available at nccn.org/patientguidelines.

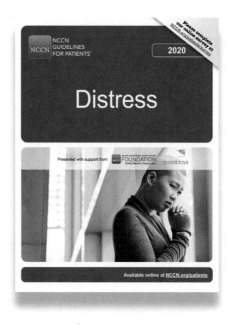

Test results

Results from blood tests, imaging studies, and biopsy will determine your treatment plan. It is important you understand what these tests mean. Ask questions and keep copies of your test results. Online patient portals are a great way to access your test results.

Whether you are going for a second opinion, test, or office visit, keep these things in mind:

➢ Bring someone with you to doctor visits. Encourage this person to ask questions and take notes. Perhaps they can record the conversation with your doctor.

➢ Write down questions and take notes during appointments. Don't be afraid to ask your care team questions. Get to know your care team and let them get to know you.

➢ Get copies of blood tests, imaging results, and reports about the specific type of cancer you have. It will be helpful when getting a second opinion.

➢ Organize your papers. Create files for insurance forms, medical records, and test results. You can do the same on your computer.

➢ Keep a list of contact information for everyone on your care team. Add it to your binder or notebook. Hang the list on your fridge or keep it by the phone.

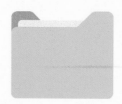

Create a medical binder

A medical binder or notebook is a great way to organize all of your records in one place.

• Make copies of blood tests, imaging results, and reports about your specific type of cancer. It will be helpful when getting a second opinion.

• Choose a binder that meets your needs. Consider a zipper pocket to include a pen, small calendar, and insurance cards.

• Create folders for insurance forms, medical records, and tests results. You can do the same on your computer.

• Use online patient portals to view your test results and other records. Download or print the records to add to your binder.

• Organize your binder in a way that works for you. Add a section for questions and to take notes.

• Bring your medical binder to appointments. You never know when you might need it!

Review

> Tests are used to find cancer, plan treatment, and check how well treatment is working.

> You will have a physical exam, including a breast exam, to see if anything feels or looks abnormal.

> Treatment can affect your fertility or your ability to have children.

> Blood tests check for signs of disease and how well organs are working.

> Imaging tests take pictures of the inside of your body.

> During a biopsy, tissue or fluid samples are removed for testing. Samples are needed to confirm the presence of cancer and to perform cancer cell tests.

> Some breast cancers have too many hormone receptors, HER2s, or both.

> A sample from a biopsy of your tumor will be tested to look for biomarkers or proteins, such as HER2.

> Genetic mutations can increase the risk of breast cancer. Your doctor might refer you for genetic testing or to speak with a genetic counselor.

3
Treatment options

29 Surgery

30 Radiation therapy

31 Endocrine therapy

33 HER2-targeted therapy

34 Chemotherapy

35 Bone-targeted therapy

36 Other targeted therapies

37 Clinical trials

38 Supportive care

39 Treatment team

40 Review

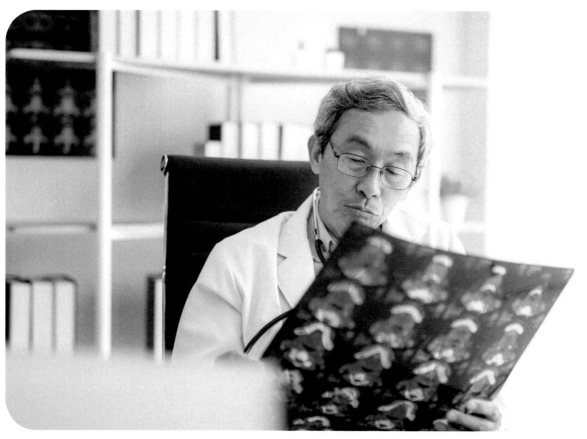

There is more than one treatment for invasive breast cancer. This chapter describes treatment options and what to expect. Not everyone will receive the same treatment. Discuss with your doctor which treatment might be best for you.

Invasive breast cancer is treatable. Treatment can be local, systemic, or a combination of both. It is important to have regular talks with your doctor about your goals for treatment and your treatment plan.

There are 2 types of treatment:

> **Local therapy** focuses on a certain area. It includes surgery, ablation, and radiation therapy.

> **Systemic therapy** works throughout the body. It includes endocrine therapy, chemotherapy, and targeted therapy.

There are many treatment options. However, not everyone will respond to treatment in the same way. Some people will do better than expected. Others will do worse. Many factors play a role in how you will respond to treatment.

Surgery

Surgery is the main or primary treatment for invasive breast cancer. Systemic therapy or radiation therapy might be used before surgery to shrink the tumor or reduce the amount of cancer (called cancer burden).

> **Preoperative** is treatment before surgery. It also called neoadjuvant therapy.

> **Postoperative** is treatment after surgery. It is also called adjuvant therapy.

Surgery requires collaboration between a breast surgeon and the reconstructive (plastic) surgeon.

Lumpectomy

Lumpectomy is the removal of abnormal cells or tumor. It is also called breast-conserving therapy. In a lumpectomy, only the tumor area along with a rim of tissue will be removed. The rest of your breast is left alone. Extra tissue is removed around the tumor to create a cancer-free area. This cancer-free area is called a surgical margin. Having a surgical margin will decrease the chance that cancer may return in that area of the breast. You may have more than one surgery to ensure all of the cancer was removed.

For invasive cancers, a lumpectomy is often done with a sentinel lymph node biopsy (SLNB). A lumpectomy might be followed by radiation therapy to part of or the whole breast. A boost is extra radiation to the tumor area.

The breast might not look the same after a lumpectomy. Speak to your doctor about how a lumpectomy might affect the look and shape of your breast and what reconstruction options are available.

Mastectomy

A total mastectomy is a surgery that removes the whole breast. Chest muscle is not removed. This operation is also called a simple mastectomy. A skin-sparing mastectomy removes the breast but not all of the skin, in order to have reconstruction. Nipple-sparing mastectomy preserves the nipple-areola complex as well. Not everyone is a candidate for nipple-sparing mastectomy.

Before removing the breast, the surgeon may do a sentinel lymph node biopsy (SLNB). Sentinel lymph nodes are the first place cancer cells are likely to have spread.

Breast reconstruction is an option after a mastectomy. It might be done at the same time as mastectomy ("immediate") or at some time following the completion of cancer treatment ("delayed"). Breast reconstruction is often done in stages.

Radiation therapy

Radiation therapy (RT) uses high-energy radiation from x-rays, gamma rays, protons, and other sources to kill cancer cells and shrink tumors. It is given over a certain period of time. Radiation therapy can be given alone or before or after surgery to treat or slow the growth of cancer. Sometimes, radiation is given with certain systemic therapies. It may be used as supportive care to help ease pain or discomfort caused by cancer.

Types of radiation therapy:

> **Whole breast radiation therapy (WBRT)** is radiation of the whole breast.

> **Accelerated partial breast irradiation (APBI)** is radiation to the area where the tumor was removed.

> **Lymph node radiation therapy** is radiation of the lymph nodes. It is also called regional nodal radiation.

Radiation may be given to the chest wall, infraclavicular region (below the collarbone), supraclavicular area (above the collarbone), lymph nodes found inside the breast (internal mammary), or axillary bed (armpit).

Endocrine therapy

The endocrine system is made up of organs and tissues that produce hormones. Hormones are natural chemicals released into the bloodstream.

There are 4 hormones that might be targeted in endocrine therapy:

> **Estrogen** is made mainly by the ovaries

> **Progesterone** is made mainly by the ovaries

> **Luteinizing hormone-releasing hormone (LHRH)** is made by a part of the brain called the hypothalamus. It tells the ovaries to make estrogen and progesterone.

> **Androgen** is made by the adrenal glands, testicles, and ovaries.

Hormones can cause breast cancer to grow. Endocrine therapy will stop your body from making hormones or it will block what hormones do in the body. This can slow tumor growth or shrink the tumor for a period of time. Endocrine therapy can be local (surgery or ablation) or systemic (drug therapy). It is sometimes called hormone therapy. It is **not** the same as hormone replacement therapy used for menopause.

The goal of endocrine therapy is to reduce the amount of estrogen or progesterone in your body.

There is one type of surgical endocrine therapy that is used for premenopausal women:

> **Bilateral oophorectomy** is surgery to remove both ovaries.

There are 5 main types of endocrine therapy:

> **Ovarian ablation** permanently stops the ovaries from making hormones. Ablation uses extreme hot or cold to stop ovaries from working.

> **Ovarian suppression** temporarily stops the ovaries from making hormones. It is achieved with drugs called LHRH agonists. These drugs stop LHRH from being made, which stops the ovaries from making hormones. LHRH agonists include goserelin (Zoladex®) and leuprolide (Lupron Depot®).

> **Aromatase inhibitors** stop a hormone called androgen from changing into estrogen by an enzyme called aromatase. They do not affect estrogen made by the ovaries. Non-steroidal aromatase inhibitors include anastrozole (Arimidex®) and letrozole (Femara®). Exemestane (Aromasin®) is a steroidal aromatase inhibitor.

> **Anti-estrogens** prevent hormones from binding to receptors. Selective estrogen receptor modulators (SERMs) block estrogen from attaching to hormone receptors. They include tamoxifen and toremifene (Fareston®). Selective estrogen receptor degraders (SERDs) block and destroy estrogen receptors. Fulvestrant (Faslodex®) is a SERD.

> **Hormones** may treat breast cancer when taken in high doses. It is not known how hormones stop breast cancer from growing. They include ethinyl estradiol, fluoxymesterone, and megestrol acetate.

Those who want to have children in the future should be referred to a fertility specialist before starting chemotherapy and/or endocrine therapy to discuss the options.

Menopause

Options for endocrine therapy are partly based on if you started or are in menopause. In menopause, the ovaries stop producing hormones and menstrual periods stop. After menopause, estrogen and progesterone levels continue to stay low.

When menstrual periods stop for 12 months or more, it is called postmenopause. If you don't get periods, a test using a blood sample may be needed to confirm your status. If you have menstrual periods, you are in premenopause.

Premenopause

In premenopause, your ovaries are the main source of estrogen and progesterone. Ovarian ablation or suppression help reduce hormone levels. For premenopause, ovarian ablation or suppression will be used with systemic therapy and/or an aromatase inhibitor.

Postmenopause

In postmenopause, your adrenal glands, liver, and body fat make small amounts of estrogen. Often in postmenopause, an aromatase inhibitor and a targeted therapy are used together.

Men with breast cancer

1 out of every 100 breast cancers occurs in men. Men with breast cancer are treated much like women. One important difference is treatment with endocrine therapy. The options are the same as for women in postmenopause. However, if men take aromatase inhibitors, they should also take a treatment to block testosterone. Aromatase inhibitors alone won't stop hormone-related cancer growth in men.

HER2-targeted therapy

HER2 is a protein involved in normal cell growth. There might be higher amounts of HER2 in your breast cancer. If this is the case, it is called HER2-positive breast cancer (HER2+). HER2-targeted therapy is drug therapy that treats HER2+ breast cancer.

HER2-targeted therapies include:

> Pertuzumab (Perjeta®)

> Trastuzumab (Herceptin®)

> Trastuzumab substitutes such as Kanjinti™, Ogivri®, Herzuma®, Ontruzant®, and Trazimera™

> Ado-trastuzumab emtansine (T-DM1) (Kadcyla®)

> Fam-trastuzumab deruxtecan-nxki (Enhertu®)

> Lapatinib (Tykerb®)

> Neratinib (Nerlynx®)

Most often, HER2-targeted therapy is given with chemotherapy. However, it might be used alone or in combination with endocrine therapy.

HER2-targeted therapies include:

> **HER2 antibodies** prevent growth signals from HER2 from outside the cell. They also increase the attack of immune cells on cancer cells. These drugs include trastuzumab (Herceptin®) and pertuzumab (Perjeta®).

> **HER2 inhibitors** stop growth signals from HER2 from within the cell. Lapatinib (Tykerb®) and neratinib (Nerlynx®) are examples of these drugs.

> **HER2 conjugates** deliver cell-specific chemotherapy. They attach to HER2s then enter the cell. Once inside, chemotherapy is released. Ado-trastuzumab emtansine (Kadcyla®) and fam-trastuzumab deruxtecan-nxki (Enhertu®) are included in this class.

Chemotherapy

Chemotherapy is a type of drug therapy used to treat cancer. Chemotherapy kills fast-growing cells throughout the body, including cancer cells and normal cells. All chemotherapy drugs affect the information inside genes called DNA (deoxyribonucleic acid). Genes tell cancer cells how and when to grow and divide. Chemotherapy disrupts the life cycle of cancer cells.

There are different types of chemotherapy used to treat invasive breast cancer:

> **Alkylating agents** damage DNA by adding a chemical to it. This group of drugs includes cyclophosphamide. Platinum-based alkylating agents contain a heavy metal that prevents cancer cells from dividing. These drugs include carboplatin and cisplatin (Platinol®).

> **Anthracyclines** damage and disrupt the making of DNA causing cell death of both cancerous and non-cancerous cells. These drugs include doxorubicin, doxorubicin liposomal injection (Doxil®), and epirubicin (Ellence®).

> **Antimetabolites** prevent the "building blocks" of DNA from being used. These drugs include capecitabine (Xeloda®), fluorouracil, gemcitabine (Gemzar®), and methotrexate.

> **Microtubule inhibitors** stop a cell from dividing into two cells. These drugs include docetaxel (Taxotere®), eribulin (Halaven™), ixabepilone (Ixempra® Kit), paclitaxel (Taxol®, Abraxane®), and vinorelbine (Navelbine®). Docetaxel, paclitaxel, and albumin-bound paclitaxel are also called taxanes.

More than one drug may be used to treat invasive breast cancer. When only one drug is used, it's called a single agent. A combination regimen is the use of two or more chemotherapy drugs.

Some chemotherapy drugs are liquids that are infused into a vein or injected under the skin with a needle. Other chemotherapy drugs may be given as a pill that is swallowed.

Most chemotherapy is given in cycles of treatment days followed by days of rest. This allows the body to recover before the next cycle. Cycles vary in length depending on which drugs are used. The number of treatment days per cycle and the total number of cycles given also varies.

Birth control during treatment

If you get pregnant during chemotherapy, radiation therapy, endocrine therapy, or systemic therapy, serious birth defects can occur. If you had menstrual periods before starting chemotherapy, use birth control without hormones. Condoms are an option. "The pill" is not. Speak to your doctor about preventing pregnancy while being treated for breast cancer.

Those who want to have children in the future should be referred to a fertility specialist before starting chemotherapy and/or endocrine therapy to discuss the options.

Bone-targeted therapy

Medicines that target the bones may be given to help relieve bone pain or reduce the risk of bone problems. Some medicines work by slowing or stopping bone breakdown, while others help increase bone thickness.

When breast cancer spreads to distant sites, it may metastasize in your bones. This puts your bones at risk for injury and disease. Such problems include bone loss (osteoporosis), fractures, bone pain, and squeezing (compression) of the spinal cord. Some treatments for breast cancer, like endocrine therapy, can cause bone loss, which put you at an increased risk for fractures.

There are 3 drugs used to prevent bone loss and fractures:

> Zoledronic acid (Zometa®)

> Pamidronate (Aredia®)

> Denosumab (Prolia®)

There are 3 drugs used to treat bone metastases:

> Zoledronic acid (Zometa®)

> Pamidronate (Aredia®)

> Denosumab (Xgeva®)

You will be screened for osteoporosis using a bone mineral density test. This measures how much calcium and other minerals are in your bones. It is also called a dual-energy x-ray absorptiometry (DEXA) scan and is painless. Bone mineral density tests look for osteoporosis and help predict your risk for bone fractures.

A baseline DEXA scan is recommended before starting endocrine therapy.

Zoledronic acid, pamidronate, and denosumab

Denosumab, pamidronate, and zoledronic acid are used to prevent bone loss (osteoporosis) and fractures caused by endocrine therapy. Denosumab and zoledronic acid are also used in those with metastatic breast cancer who have bone metastases to help prevent fractures or spinal cord compression. You might have blood tests to monitor kidney function, calcium levels, and magnesium levels. A calcium and vitamin D supplement will be recommended by your doctor.

Let your dentist know if you are taking any of these medicines. Also, ask your doctor how these medicines might affect your teeth and jaw. Osteonecrosis, or bone tissue death of the jaw, is a rare but serious side effect. Tell your doctor about any planned trips to the dentist. It will be important to take care of your teeth and to see a dentist before starting treatment with any of these drugs.

Other targeted therapies

CDK4/6 inhibitors

Cyclin-dependent kinase (CDK) is a cell protein that helps cells grow and divide. For hormone-positive, HER2- cancer, taking a CDK4/6 inhibitor with endocrine therapy may help control cancer longer. With all CDK4/6 regimens, premenopausal women must also receive ovarian ablation or suppression.

mTOR inhibitors

mTOR is a cell protein that helps cells grow and divide. Endocrine therapy may stop working if mTOR becomes overactive. mTOR inhibitors are used to get endocrine therapy working again.

Everolimus (Afinitor®) is an mTOR inhibitor. Most often, it is taken with exemestane. For some, it may be taken with fulvestrant or tamoxifen.

PARP inhibitors

Cancer cells often become damaged. PARP is a cell protein that repairs cancer cells and allows them to survive. Blocking PARP can cause cancer cells to die. Olaparib (Lynparza®) and talazoparib (Talzenna®) are PARP inhibitors. You must have the *BRCA1* or *BRCA2* mutation and your breast cancer must be HER2- for PARP inhibitors to be effective.

PIK3CA inhibitor

The *PIK3CA* gene is one of the most frequently mutated genes in breast cancers. A mutation in this gene can lead to increased growth of cancer cells and resistance to various treatments.

You should not become pregnant during treatment with radiation therapy or systemic therapy.

Immunotherapy

Immunotherapy is a type of systemic treatment that increases the activity of your immune system. By doing so, it improves your body's ability to find and destroy cancer cells. Immunotherapy can be given alone or with other types of treatment.

Clinical trials

Clinical trials study how safe and helpful tests and treatments are for people. Clinical trials find out how to prevent, diagnose, and treat a disease like cancer. Because of clinical trials, doctors find safe and helpful ways to improve your care and treatment of cancer.

Clinical trials have 4 phases.

Phase I trials aim to find the safest and best dose of a new drug. Another aim is to find the best way to give the drug with the fewest side effects.

Phase II trials assess if a drug works for a specific type of cancer.

Phase III trials compare a new drug to a standard treatment.

Phase IV trials evaluate a drug's safety and treatment results after it has been approved.

To join a clinical trial, you must meet the conditions of the study. Patients in a clinical trial often are alike in terms of their cancer and general health. This helps to ensure that any change is from the treatment and not because of differences between patients.

If you decide to join a clinical trial, you will need to review and sign a paper called an informed consent form. This form describes the study in detail, including the risks and benefits. Even after you sign a consent form, you can stop taking part in a clinical trial at any time.

Ask your treatment team if there is an open clinical trial that you can join. There may be clinical trials where you're getting treatment or

Finding a clinical trial

- Search the National Institutes of Health (NIH) database for clinical trials. It includes publicly and privately funded clinical trials, whom to contact, and how to enroll. Look for an open clinical trial for your specific type of cancer. Go to **ClinicalTrials.gov**.

- The National Cancer Institute's Cancer Information Service (CIS) provides up-to-date information on clinical trials. You can call, e-mail, or chat live. Call 1.800.4.CANCER (800.422.6237) or go to **cancer.gov**.

at other treatment centers nearby. Discuss the risks and benefits of joining a clinical trial with your care team. Together, decide if a clinical trial is right for you.

NCCN experts encourage patients to join a clinical trial when it is the best option for the patient.

Supportive care

Supportive care is health care that relieves symptoms caused by cancer or its treatment and improves quality of life. It might include pain relief (palliative care), emotional or spiritual support, financial aid, or family counseling. Tell your care team how you are feeling and about any side effects.

Treatment side effects

All cancer treatments can cause unwanted health issues. Such health issues are called side effects. Side effects depend on many factors. These factors include the drug type and dose, length of treatment, and the person. Some side effects may be harmful to your health. Others may just be unpleasant.

Ask for a complete list of side effects of your treatments. Also, tell your treatment team about any new or worsening symptoms. There may be ways to help you feel better. There are also ways to prevent some side effects.

Trouble eating

Sometimes side effects from surgery, cancer, or its treatment might cause you to feel not hungry or sick to your stomach (nauseated). You might have a sore mouth. Healthy eating is important during treatment. It includes eating a balanced diet, eating the right amount of food, and drinking enough fluids. A registered dietitian who is an expert in nutrition and food can help. Speak to your care team if you have trouble eating.

For more information, read the *NCCN Guidelines for Patients®: Nausea and Vomiting,* available at nccn.org/patientguidelines

Lymphedema

Lymphedema is a condition in which extra lymph fluid builds up in tissues and causes swelling. It may occur when part of the lymph system is damaged or blocked, such as during surgery to remove lymph nodes, or radiation therapy. Cancers that block lymph vessels can also cause lymphedema. Swelling usually develops slowly over time. It may develop during treatment or it may start years after treatment. If you have lymphedema, you may be referred to an expert in lymphedema management. The swelling may be reduced by exercise, massage, compression sleeves, and other means. Ask your care team about the ways to treat lymphedema.

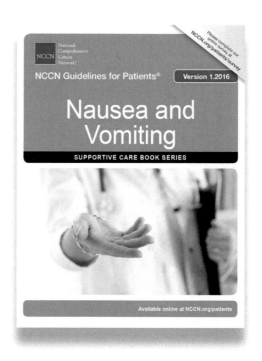

Treatment team

Treating breast cancer takes a team approach. Some members of your care team will be with you throughout cancer treatment, while others will only be there for parts of it. Get to know your care team and let them get to know you.

> **Your primary care doctor** handles medical care not related to your cancer. This person can help you express your feelings about treatments to your cancer care team.

> **A pathologist** reads tests and studies the cells, tissues, and organs removed during a biopsy or surgery.

> **A diagnostic radiologist** reads the results of x-rays and other imaging tests.

> **A surgical oncologist** performs operations to remove cancer.

> **A medical oncologist** treats cancer in adults using systemic therapy. Often, this person will lead the overall treatment team and keep track of tests and exams done by other specialists. A medical oncologist will often coordinate your care. Ask who will coordinate your care.

> **A palliative care specialist** is an expert in the treatment of symptoms caused by the cancer with the goal of improving a patient's quality of life and easing suffering.

> **Advanced practice providers** are an important part of any team. These are registered nurse practitioners and physician assistants who monitor your health and provide care.

> **Oncology nurses** provide your hands-on care, like giving systemic therapy, managing your care, answering questions, and helping you cope with side effects.

> **Nutritionists** can provide guidance on what foods or diet are most suitable for your particular condition.

> **Psychologists and psychiatrists** are mental health experts who can help manage issues such as depression, anxiety, or other mental health conditions that can affect how you feel.

Depending on your diagnosis, your team might include:

> **An anesthesiologist** who gives anesthesia, a medicine so you do not feel pain during surgery or procedures

> **An interventional radiologist** who performs needle biopsies of tumors and sometimes performs ablation therapies or places ports for treatment

> **A radiation oncologist** who prescribes and plans radiation therapy to treat cancer

> **A plastic surgeon** who performs breast reconstruction for those undergoing mastectomy, if desired

> **An occupational therapist** who helps people with the tasks of daily living

> **A physical therapist** who helps people move with greater comfort and ease

> **A certified lymphedema therapist** who gives a type of massage called manual lymph drainage

You know your body better than anyone. Help other team members understand:

> How you feel

> What you need

> What is working and what is not

Keep a list of names and contact information for each member of your team. This will make it easier for you and anyone involved in your care to know whom to contact with questions or concerns.

> Get to know your care team and let them get to know you.

Review

> Invasive breast cancer is treatable. The goal of treatment is to remove the tumor, when possible, and prevent or slow the spread of cancer.

> Local therapy focuses on a certain area. It includes surgery, ablation, and radiation therapy.

> Systemic therapy works throughout the body. It includes endocrine therapy, chemotherapy, and targeted therapy.

> Targeted therapies can block the ways cancer cells grow, divide, and move in the body.

> Treatment for invasive breast cancer is a combination of therapies.

> Those who want to have children in the future should be referred to a fertility specialist before starting chemotherapy and/or endocrine therapy to discuss the options.

> A clinical trial is a type of research that studies a treatment to see how safe it is and how well it works.

> Supportive care is health care that relieves symptoms caused by cancer or cancer treatment and improves quality of life.

4
Breast reconstruction

42   Volume displacement

42   Implants and flaps

43   Nipple replacement

43   Review

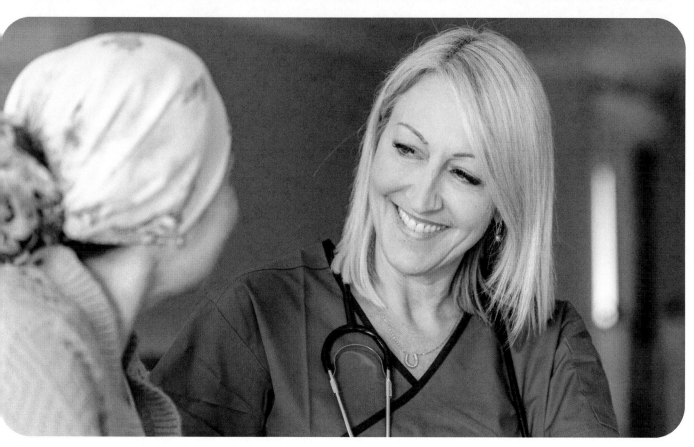

Breast reconstruction is surgery to rebuild the shape and look of the breast. In many cases, breast reconstruction involves a staged approach. It might require more than one procedure. This chapter offers more information on breast reconstruction.

Volume displacement

If you will have a lumpectomy, your breast can be re-shaped. This procedure is called volume displacement. It is often done by the cancer surgeon right after the lumpectomy. The surgeon will shift the remaining breast tissue to fill the gap left by the removed tumor.

If volume displacement is planned, a larger piece of your breast will need to be removed. Despite a larger piece being removed, the natural look of your breast will be kept.

You may not like the results of the volume displacement. In this case, breast revision surgery may help. This surgery is done by a plastic surgeon. A second volume displacement may be an option, too. A third option is to get breast implants or flaps, which are described next.

Implants and flaps

Breasts can be reconstructed with implants and flaps. All methods are generally safe, but as with any surgery, there are risks. Ask your treatment team for a complete list of side effects.

You may have a choice as to when breast reconstruction is done. Immediate reconstruction is finished within hours after removing the breast. Delayed reconstruction can occur months or years after the cancer surgery. A plastic surgeon performs breast reconstruction.

Implants
Breast implants are small bags filled with salt water, silicone gel, or both. They are placed under the breast skin or muscle. A balloon-like device, called an expander, may be used first to stretch out tissue. It will be placed under your skin or muscle and enlarged every few weeks for two to three months.

Implants have a small risk of leaking. You may feel pain from the implant or expander. Scar tissue or tissue death can occur.

Flaps
Breasts can be remade using tissue from your body, known as "flaps." Flaps are taken from the belly area, butt, or from under the shoulder blade. Some flaps are completely removed and then sewn in place. Other flaps stay attached but are slid over and sewn into place.

Flaps can cause problems. There may be tissue death. Death of fat cells may cause lumps. A hernia may occur from muscle weakness. Problems are more likely to occur among those who have diabetes or smoke.

Implants and flaps

Some breasts are reconstructed with both implants and flaps. This method may give the reconstructed breast more volume to match the other breast. For any reconstruction, you may need surgery on your other breast to match the two breasts in size and shape.

Nipple replacement

Like your breast, you can have your nipple remade. To rebuild a nipple, a plastic surgeon can use surrounding tissues. Also, nipples can be remade with tissue from the thigh, other nipple, or the sex organs between your legs (vulva). Tissue can be darkened with a tattoo to look more like a nipple.

Review

- > Breast reconstruction is surgery to rebuild the shape and look of the breast.

- > Volume displacement is a shifting of the breast tissue to fill the hole left by a lumpectomy.

- > Breasts that are fully removed can be remade with breast implants, flaps, or both.

- > Removed nipples can be remade with body tissue.

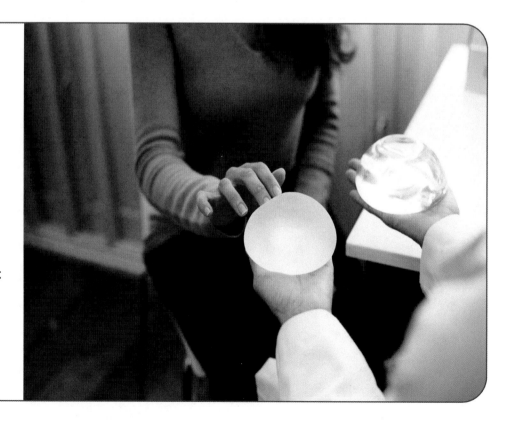

Breast implants

Breast implants are one method of reconstructing breasts. They are small bags filled with salt water, silicone gel, or both. They are placed under the breast skin and muscle.

5
Stage 1, 2, and 3A

45 Testing

46 Surgery options

48 Adjuvant treatment

57 Follow-up care

58 Review

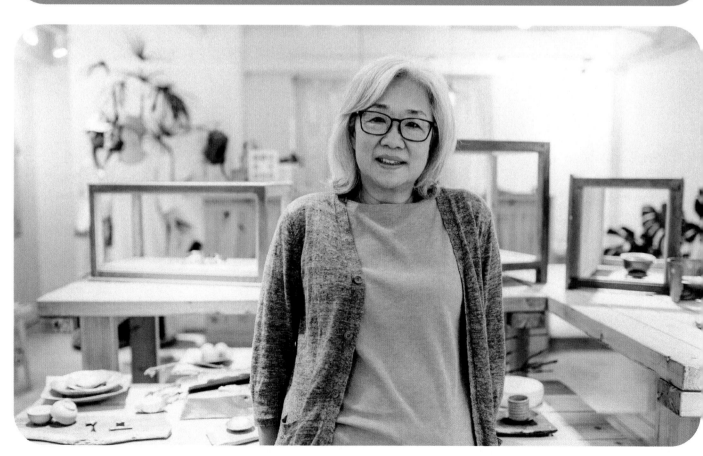

Surgery is the main or primary treatment for invasive breast cancer. Treatment before surgery is called preoperative therapy. Not all cancers need treatment before surgery. This chapter is for those who will not have preoperative therapy. Together, you and your doctor will choose the best option for you.

Not all cancers need treatment before surgery. If your doctor is considering treatment before surgery (preoperative), then Chapter 6 is where you can find that information. This chapter is for those who will not have preoperative therapy.

Testing

If your doctor feels your cancer does not need systemic therapy or radiation therapy before surgery, then you will have the tests found in Guide 2.

Guide 2
Testing: Not a candidate for preoperative systemic therapy

Needed	• Medical history and physical exam • Diagnostic mammogram • Determine tumor ER/PR and HER2 status • Genetic counseling if at risk for hereditary breast cancer • Fertility counseling • Pregnancy test • Screen for distress
Other	• Ultrasound of breast • Breast MRI • CBC and comprehensive metabolic panel (including liver function tests and alkaline phosphatase) • Bone scan or sodium fluoride PET/CT • CT with contrast of abdomen with or without pelvis or MRI with contrast • Chest CT with contrast (for diagnosis if have lung symptoms) • FDG PET/CT

Surgery options

There are 2 surgery options:

> Lumpectomy

> Total mastectomy

Both options include axillary lymph node staging. Radiation therapy (RT) often follows surgery. When chemotherapy is given, radiation often follows.

Lumpectomy with ALN staging

A lumpectomy is surgery to remove a tumor in the breast. Treatment after a lumpectomy is based on the type of cancer and if cancer is found in the axillary lymph nodes (ALNs). It is usually radiation therapy (RT). Chemotherapy might be given before RT. If cancer is found in the lymph nodes, then RT to the whole breast is given. This is called whole breast radiation therapy (WBRT). If no cancer was found in the lymph nodes, then radiation to the area where the cancer was removed or accelerated partial breast irradiation (APBI) may be given. See Guide 3.

Guide 3
Treatment options: Lumpectomy with axillary lymph node staging

4 or more positive axillary nodes	• Whole breast radiation therapy (WBRT) • WBRT with boost to tumor bed, infraclavicular region, supraclavicular area, internal mammary nodes, and any part of the axillary bed at risk. • It is common for radiation to follow chemotherapy (if given).
1 to 3 positive axillary nodes	• WBRT • WBRT with boost to tumor bed. Strongly consider radiation therapy (RT) to infraclavicular region, supraclavicular area, internal mammary nodes, and any part of the axillary bed at risk. • It is common for RT to follow chemotherapy (if given).
Negative axillary nodes	• RT with or without boost to tumor bed, and consider regional nodal irradiation in some cases. • Consider accelerated partial breast irradiation (APBI) in some low-risk patients. • It is common for RT to follow chemotherapy when chemotherapy is given.

Total mastectomy

A total mastectomy is a surgery that removes the whole breast and some lymph nodes. Treatment after a mastectomy is based on if cancer was found in the axillary lymph nodes and the number of lymph nodes that tested positive. Treatment is usually radiation therapy (RT). Chemotherapy might be given before RT. If there is a positive surgical margin, there may be cancer remaining after surgery. In this case, you might have more surgery to remove the cancer. See Guide 4.

Guide 4
Treatment options: Total mastectomy with axillary lymph node staging

4 or more positive axillary nodes	• Consider diagnostic CT of chest/abdomen and pelvis with contrast, bone scan, and FDG PET/CT. • Radiation therapy to chest wall and infraclavicular region, supraclavicular area, internal mammary nodes, and any part of the axillary bed at risk. • It is common for RT to follow chemotherapy when chemotherapy is given.
1 to 3 positive axillary nodes	• Strongly consider RT to chest wall and infraclavicular region, supraclavicular area, internal mammary nodes, and any part of the axillary bed at risk. • It is common for RT to follow chemotherapy when chemotherapy is given.
Negative axillary nodes and tumor is more than 5 cm	• Consider RT to chest wall alone or with any of the following: infraclavicular region, supraclavicular area, internal mammary nodes, and any part of the axillary bed at risk. • It is common for RT to follow chemotherapy when chemotherapy is given.
Positive surgical margin	• More surgery to achieve negative margins is preferred. If not possible, then strongly consider RT to chest wall alone or with any of the following: infraclavicular region, supraclavicular area, internal mammary nodes, and any part of the axillary bed at risk. • It is common for RT to follow chemotherapy when chemotherapy is given.
Negative axillary nodes and tumor is 5 cm or less	• If surgical margin is less than 1 mm, then consider RT to chest wall alone or with regional nodal radiation in some cases. • It is common for RT to follow chemotherapy when chemotherapy is given. • If surgical margin is 1 mm or more, then no radiation therapy in most cases.

Adjuvant treatment

Treatment after surgery is called adjuvant treatment. It is based on the pathologic stage and the tumor histology. After surgery, a pathologist will examine the removed tissue and determine the pathologic stage. An example of a tumor stage after surgery might be pT2. Lymph node micrometastases are written as pN1mi. Ipsilateral means on the same side of the body.

Adjuvant systemic therapy is given after surgery to kill any remaining cancer cells and to help reduce the risk of cancer returning. This treatment is based on histology and hormone receptor status. Histology is the study of the anatomy (structure) of cells, tissues, and organs under a microscope. Depending on the histology, HER2 status may be a factor. If cancer is hormone-positive (ER+ and/or PR+) and HER2-, then oncologists also take into account if there is cancer in lymph nodes called node positive (node+).

Systemic therapies might be used alone or in combination. Ask your medical oncologist why one treatment might be preferred over another for your type of cancer.

For treatment by histology and hormone receptor status see Guide 5.

Guide 5
Treatment by histology and hormone receptor status

Histology type:

- **Ductal/NST**
- **Lobular**
- **Mixed**
- **Micropapillary**
- **Metaplastic**

- ER+ and/or PR+ with HER2+ see Guide 6
- ER+ and/or PR+ with HER2- and node- see Guide 7
- ER+ and/or PR+ with HER2- and node+ see Guide 8
- ER- and PR- with HER2+ see Guide 10
- ER- and PR- with HER2- (triple negative) see Guide 11

Favorable histology type:

- **Pure tubular**
- **Pure mucinous**
- **Pure cribriform**
- **Encapsulated or solid papillary carcinoma**
- **Other rare forms**

- ER+ and/or PR+ see Guide 13
- ER- and PR- see Guide 13

ER+ and/or PR+ with HER2+

In hormone-positive cancer, estrogen (ER+) and/or progesterone receptors (PR+) are found. When HER2 receptors are found, it is also HER2+. This cancer is sometimes called triple-positive breast cancer. Endocrine therapy is used to treat hormone-positive breast cancer. Chemotherapy with a HER2-targeted therapy is used to treat HER2+ cancer.

Examples of HER2-targeted therapy used after surgery include trastuzumab and pertuzumab. Systemic therapies might be used alone or in combination. Ask your medical oncologist why one treatment might be preferred over another for your type of cancer.

Systemic adjuvant treatment options for ER+ and/or PR+ with HER2+ are found in Guide 6.

Guide 6
Systemic adjuvant treatment options: ER+ and/or PR+ with HER2+

Histology type:

- Ductal/NST
- Lobular
- Mixed
- Micropapillary

pT1, pT2, or pT3; and pN0 or pN1mi (axillary node metastasis of 2 mm or less)

If tumor of 0.5 cm or less and pN0, consider:
- Endocrine therapy
- Endocrine therapy and chemotherapy with trastuzumab

If tumor of 0.5 cm or less and pN1mi, consider:
- Endocrine therapy
- Chemotherapy with trastuzumab and endocrine therapy

If tumor is 0.6 to 1.0 cm:
- Chemotherapy with trastuzumab and endocrine therapy

If tumor larger than 1 cm:
- Chemotherapy with trastuzumab, pertuzumab, and endocrine therapy

Node positive (1 or more ipsilateral metastases larger than 2 mm)
- Chemotherapy with trastuzumab and endocrine therapy
- Chemotherapy with trastuzumab, pertuzumab, and endocrine therapy

ER+ and/or PR+ with HER2- and node-

In hormone-positive cancer, estrogen (ER+) and/or progesterone receptors (PR+) are found. Endocrine therapy is used to treat hormone-positive breast cancer. Endocrine therapy might be used alone or after chemotherapy. Since there are no HER2 receptors, therapy targeting the HER2 receptors is not used. Often, chemotherapy is used instead. When no cancer is found in the lymph nodes, it is node negative (node-).

A gene tumor test might be done. It would be used to determine if there is benefit from chemotherapy. Ask your doctor if you will have a gene test and what your score means.

Systemic adjuvant treatment options for ER+ and/or PR+ with HER2- and node- are found in Guide 7.

Guide 7
Systemic adjuvant treatment options: ER+ and/or PR+ with HER2- and node-

Histology type:

- **Ductal/NST**
- **Lobular**
- **Mixed**
- **Micropapillary**

pT1, pT2, or pT3; and pN0 →

If tumor of 0.5 cm or less and pN0, consider:
- Endocrine therapy

If tumor larger than 0.5 cm and gene test not done:
- Endocrine therapy
- Chemotherapy followed by endocrine therapy

If tumor larger than 0.5 cm and recurrence score is less than 26:
- Endocrine therapy

If tumor larger than 0.5 cm and recurrence score is 26 to 30:
- Endocrine therapy
- Chemotherapy followed by endocrine therapy

If tumor larger than 0.5 cm and recurrence score is 31 or more:
- Chemotherapy followed by endocrine therapy

ER+ and/or PR+ with HER2- and node+

In hormone-positive cancer, estrogen (ER+) and/or progesterone receptors (PR+) are found. Endocrine therapy is used to treat hormone-positive breast cancer. Endocrine therapy might be used alone or after chemotherapy. Chemotherapy is used when HER2 is negative. Since there are no HER2 receptors, targeted therapy is not used. When there is cancer in the lymph nodes, it is node positive (node+).

A gene tumor test might be done. It would be used to predict the benefit from chemotherapy. Ask your doctor if you will have a gene test and what your results mean.

Systemic adjuvant treatment options for ER+ and/or PR+ with HER2- and node+ are found in Guide 8.

Guide 8
Systemic adjuvant treatment options: ER+ and/or PR+ with HER2- and node+

Histology type:		
• Ductal/NST • Lobular • Mixed • Micropapillary	• pN1mi (axillary node metastasis of 2 mm or less) or • N1 (less than 4 nodes) ➡	**If chemotherapy not an option:** • Endocrine therapy **If chemotherapy an option and gene test available:** • Endocrine therapy • Chemotherapy followed endocrine therapy **If chemotherapy an option, but gene test not available:** • Chemotherapy followed by endocrine therapy
	Node positive (4 or more ipsilateral metastases larger than 2 mm) ➡	• Chemotherapy followed by endocrine therapy

ER- and/or PR- with HER2+

In hormone-negative cancer, there are no receptors for estrogen (ER-) and progesterone (PR-). When HER2 receptors are found, it is HER2-positive (HER2+). Since this cancer is hormone negative, treatment will focus on targeting HER2.

HER2-targeted therapy options can be found in Guide 9.

Guide 9
Systemic therapy for HER2+

Preferred options	• Doxorubicin and cyclophosphamide followed by paclitaxel with trastuzumab • Doxorubicin and cyclophosphamide followed by paclitaxel with trastuzumab and pertuzumab • Paclitaxel with trastuzumab • Docetaxel, carboplatin, and trastuzumab (TCH) • Docetaxel, carboplatin, trastuzumab, and pertuzumab (TCHP)
Useful in some cases	• Docetaxel with cyclophosphamide and trastuzumab
Other recommended	• Doxorubicin with cyclophosphamide followed by docetaxel with trastuzumab • Doxorubicin with cyclophosphamide followed by docetaxel with trastuzumab and pertuzumab

Systemic adjuvant treatment options for ER- and/or PR- with HER2+ are found in Guide 10.

Guide 10
Systemic adjuvant treatment options: ER- and PR- with HER2+

Histology type:	pT1, pT2, or pT3; and pN0 or pN1mi (axillary node metastasis of 2 mm or less)	If tumor of 0.5 cm or less and pN0, consider: • Chemotherapy with trastuzumab
• Ductal/NST • Lobular • Mixed • Micropapillary		If tumor of 0.5 cm or less and pN1mi, consider: • Chemotherapy with trastuzumab
		If tumor is 0.6 to 1.0 cm, consider: • Chemotherapy with trastuzumab
		If tumor larger than 1 cm: • Chemotherapy with trastuzumab
	Node positive (1 or more ipsilateral metastases larger than 2 mm)	• Chemotherapy with trastuzumab • Chemotherapy with trastuzumab and pertuzumab

Triple-negative breast cancer

In triple-negative breast cancer (TNBC), receptors for estrogen, progesterone, and HER2 are not found. This means that the breast cancer cells have tested negative for HER2, estrogen hormone receptors, and progesterone hormone receptors. Since there are no HER2 receptors, HER2-targeted therapy is not an option. And since there are no estrogen or progesterone hormone receptors, endocrine therapy is not an option.

Systemic adjuvant treatment options for TNBC are found in Guide 11.

Guide 11
Systemic adjuvant treatment options: ER- and PR- with HER2- (TNBC)

Histology type:	pT1, pT2, or pT3; and pN0 or pN1mi (axillary node metastasis of 2 mm or less)	If tumor is 0.5 cm or less and pN0: • No adjuvant therapy • Chemotherapy may be considered if high-risk features
• Ductal/NST • Lobular • Mixed • Micropapillary • Metaplastic		If tumor is 0.5 cm or less and pN1mi, consider: • Chemotherapy
		If tumor is 0.6 to 1.0 cm, consider: • Chemotherapy
		If tumor larger than 1 cm: • Chemotherapy
	Node positive (1 or more ipsilateral metastases larger than 2 mm)	• Chemotherapy

Since this cancer is hormone negative and HER2-, treatment will likely be chemotherapy as found in Guide 12.

Guide 12
Systemic therapy for HER2-

Preferred options	• Doxorubicin and cyclophosphamide followed by paclitaxel • Docetaxel and cyclophosphamide (TC)
Useful in some cases	• Doxorubicin with cyclophosphamide • Cyclophosphamide, methotrexate, and fluorouracil (CMF) • Doxorubicin with cyclophosphamide followed by paclitaxel
Other recommended	• Doxorubicin and cyclophosphamide followed by docetaxel • Epirubicin and cyclophosphamide (EC) • Docetaxel, doxorubicin, and cyclophosphamide (TAC)

Favorable histologies

A favorable histology is one that has a favorable or good prognosis. A prognosis is the path your cancer will likely take. These tumors might respond better to treatment than other tumors. They also might have less risk of returning. Treatment for favorable histologies that are HER2- can be found in Guide 13.

Guide 13
Treatment for favorable histologies

ER+ and/or PR+ with HER2- • **Pure tubular** • **Pure mucinous** • **Pure cribriform** • **Encapsulated or solid papillary carcinoma**	pT1, pT2, or pT3; and pN0 or pN1mi (axillary node metastasis of 2 mm or less) ➡	If tumor is less than 1 cm, consider: • Endocrine therapy to reduce future risk If tumor is 1 to 2.9 cm, consider: • Endocrine therapy If tumor is 3 cm or more: • Endocrine therapy
	Node positive (1 or more ipsilateral metastases larger than 2 mm) ➡	• Endocrine therapy alone or with adjuvant chemotherapy
ER- and PR- with HER2- • **Adenoid cystic carcinoma** • **Salivary secretory carcinoma** • **Other rare types**		• Consider systemic therapy only in node+ (positive) disease

Follow-up care

After treatment, you will enter follow-up care. During this time, your health will be monitored for side effects of treatment and the return of cancer. This is part of your survivorship care plan.

It is important to keep follow-up visits and tests. Tell your doctor about any symptoms such as headaches or bone pain. Continue to take all medicine such as endocrine therapy exactly as prescribed and do not miss or skip doses. You should receive a personalized survivorship care plan. It will provide a summary of possible long-term effects of treatment and list follow-up tests. Find out how your primary care provider will coordinate with specialists for your follow-up care.

Follow-up care can be found in Guide 14.

Guide 14
Follow-up care

Medical history and physical exam 1 to 4 times per year as needed for 5 years, then every year

Periodic screening for changes in family history

Genetic testing and referral to genetic counseling as needed

Monitor for lymphedema and refer for lymphedema management as needed

Mammogram every 12 months (not needed on reconstructed breast)

If signs and symptoms of metastases, then blood and imaging tests

If on endocrine therapy, continue to take endocrine therapy. Do not miss or skip doses.

Those with uterus and are on tamoxifen should have a gynecology exam every 12 months

Those on an aromatase inhibitor or who later have ovarian failure should have bone density tests

Maintain an ideal weight, be active, eat a healthy diet, exercise, limit alcohol, and quit smoking

Review

> Surgery is the main or primary treatment for invasive breast cancer. Radiation therapy (RT) often follows surgery. If you have chemotherapy, RT is given after chemotherapy.

> Treatment after surgery is called adjuvant treatment. It is based on the pathologic stage. During surgery, your tumor is tested to determine the pathologic stage.

> Adjuvant systemic therapy is given after surgery to kill any remaining cancer cells and to help prevent the return of cancer.

> Adjuvant treatment is based on the stage, histology, and hormone receptor status. Histology is the study of the anatomy (structure) of cells, tissues, and organs under a microscope.

> A favorable histology is one that has a favorable or good prognosis.

> In hormone-positive cancer, estrogen (ER+) and/or progesterone receptors (PR+) are found.

> In triple-negative breast cancer (TNBC), receptors for estrogen, progesterone, and HER2 are not found.

> It is important to keep follow-up visits and tests. Continue to take all medicines as prescribed.

6
Stage 3

60   Overview

61   Testing

62   Tumor is operable

64   Tumor is inoperable

64   Adjuvant treatment

69   Follow-up care

70   Review

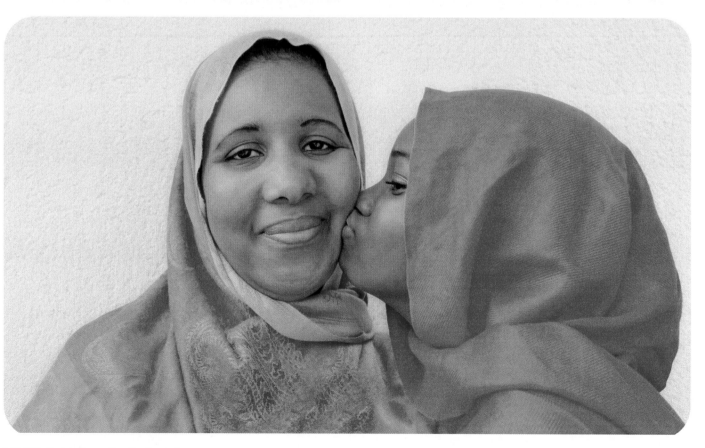

In stage 3 breast cancer, the cancer can be large and in the lymph nodes, the lymph nodes can be fixed (or not moveable), or the cancer can involve the skin or chest wall. The goal of treatment is to shrink the tumor or amount of cancer before surgery. Treatment before surgery is called preoperative or neoadjuvant therapy. It can be systemic therapy or radiation therapy. Preoperative therapy is not for everyone. Together, you and your doctor will choose the best option for you.

Overview

This chapter is for those who have stage 3 breast cancer or for those who would benefit from treatment before surgery. Treatment before surgery is called preoperative or neoadjuvant therapy. In stage 3 breast cancer, the cancer can be large and in the lymph nodes, the lymph nodes can be fixed (or not moveable), or the cancer can involve the skin or chest wall. It is not metastatic.

Treatment before surgery is called preoperative. It can be systemic (drug) therapy or radiation therapy. Preoperative systemic therapy has benefits.

It can:

> Help preserve the breast

> Shrink the tumor

> Shrink the tumor so it can be removed with surgery

> Provide important information about how your tumor responds to therapy, which is very helpful in those with triple-negative (TNBC) and HER2+ breast cancer

> Help choose adjuvant regimens in those with HER2+ and TNBC with residual disease

> Allow time for genetic testing

> Allow time to plan breast reconstruction in those choosing mastectomy

> Allow time for fewer lymph nodes to be removed at the time of surgery

There are risks with any treatment. Cancer can still progress during preoperative systemic therapy.

Testing

Not everyone will benefit from preoperative therapy. If preoperative systemic therapy is an option for you, then you will have tests before starting treatment. These tests will determine if your cancer can be removed with surgery (operable) or cannot be removed with surgery at this time (inoperable). Testing can be found in Guide 15.

Guide 15
Tests before starting preoperative systemic therapy

Needed	• Medical history and physical exam • Diagnostic mammogram • Axillary lymph node exam • Determine tumor ER/PR and HER2 status • Genetic counseling if at risk for hereditary breast cancer • Fertility counseling if premenopausal • Pregnancy test if premenopausal • Screen for distress
Other	• Ultrasound of breast • Ultrasound of axillary lymph nodes • Biopsy of lymph nodes suspected of cancer • CBC and comprehensive metabolic panel (including liver function tests and alkaline phosphatase) • Chest CT with contrast (for diagnosis) • CT with contrast of abdomen with or without pelvis or MRI with contrast • Bone scan or sodium fluoride PET/CT, if needed • FDG PET/CT • Breast MRI

Tumor is operable

You will have the following additional tests or procedures before starting preoperative systemic therapy, if not done before:

> Core biopsy of breast

> The placement of clips - The clips are placed to help the surgeon know where to operate in case the cancer goes away with preoperative therapy. Clips are placed at the time of surgery for radiation planning.

> Axillary lymph node ultrasound or MRI

> Biopsy of suspicious lymph nodes

> An sentinel lymph node biopsy (SLNB) might be done

Preoperative therapy is based on hormone receptor (HR) and HER2 status. For systemic therapy options for HER2+ cancer, see Guide 16.

Guide 16 Systemic therapy for HER2+	
Preferred options	• Doxorubicin and cyclophosphamide followed by paclitaxel with trastuzumab • Doxorubicin and cyclophosphamide followed by paclitaxel with trastuzumab and pertuzumab • Paclitaxel with trastuzumab • Docetaxel, carboplatin, and trastuzumab (TCH) • Docetaxel, carboplatin, trastuzumab, and pertuzumab (TCHP) • If no residual disease after preoperative therapy or no preoperative therapy: Complete up to one year of HER2-targeted therapy with trastuzumab alone or with pertuzumab • If residual disease after preoperative therapy: Ado-trastuzumab emtansine alone. If ado-trastuzumab emtansine discontinued for toxicity, then trastuzumab alone or with pertuzumab to complete one year of therapy.
Useful in some cases	• Docetaxel with cyclophosphamide and trastuzumab
Other recommended	• Doxorubicin with cyclophosphamide followed by docetaxel with trastuzumab • Doxorubicin with cyclophosphamide followed by docetaxel with trastuzumab and pertuzumab

Surgery

Surgery options depend on how your cancer responded to preoperative therapy. A complete response means there is no evidence of cancer. In a partial response, the tumor in the breast or lymph nodes has shrunk in size.

A lumpectomy or mastectomy are options depending on the size and location of the tumor. Systemic therapy and radiation therapy may follow surgery. See Guide 17.

Guide 17
Surgery and adjuvant treatment based on response to preoperative treatment

Complete response or Partial response (lumpectomy possible)

Lumpectomy with surgical axillary lymph node staging followed by
- Systemic therapy (see Guide 19) and
- Radiation therapy

Clinical N1 and ypN0:
- Adjuvant radiation therapy (RT) to the whole breast with or without boost to the tumor bed; and strongly consider radiation to the supraclavicular/infraclavicular region and area, internal mammary nodes, and any part of the axillary bed at risk

Any ypN+:
- Adjuvant RT to the whole breast (with or without boost to the tumor bed) includes the supraclavicular/infraclavicular region and area, internal mammary nodes, and any part of the axillary bed at risk

Partial response (lumpectomy not possible) or Confirmed disease progression at any time (lumpectomy not possible)

Mastectomy with surgical axillary lymph node staging and optional breast reconstruction followed by
- Systemic therapy (see Guide19) and
- Radiation therapy

Clinical N1 and ypN0:
- Strongly consider RT to the chest wall, supraclavicular/infraclavicular regions, internal mammary nodes, and any part of the axillary bed at risk

Any ypN:
- RT to the chest wall and supraclavicular/infraclavicular regions, internal mammary nodes, and any part of the axillary bed at risk

Tumor is inoperable

If initial tests show the tumor cannot be removed with surgery (inoperable), then you will have preoperative therapy. During and after preoperative therapy, you will have tests to monitor treatment. If the tumor shrinks or the cancer burden is reduced, then surgery might be possible. If the tumor did not shrink enough to be removed with surgery, then you will have more preoperative therapy. Talk with your doctor about what types of preoperative therapy are right for you. See Guide 18.

Adjuvant treatment

Many people have treatment after surgery. Treatment after surgery is called adjuvant therapy. Adjuvant therapy is based on the size of the tumor, if cancer remains (residual disease), and if cancer in the lymph nodes is found. A complete response means there is no evidence of cancer.

Your tumor will be restaged after preoperative therapy. Staging will be done by looking at tissue removed during surgery. This is called the pathologic stage or surgical stage. It might look like this: ypT0N0. The "y" means you had therapy before surgery.

ER+ and/or PR+ is called hormone positive. It is often treated with adjuvant endocrine therapy. HER2-targeted therapy is often used to treat HER2+ cancer. Systemic therapies might be used alone or in combination. Ask your

---

Guide 18   BINV-14
Treatment options based on preoperative treatment response

Tumor shrunk and surgery is possible	• Mastectomy with surgical axillary lymph node staging and optional breast reconstruction • Lumpectomy with surgical axillary lymph node staging	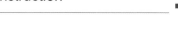	Adjuvant systemic therapy (see Guide 19) and adjuvant RT to the whole breast or chest wall, supraclavicular/infraclavicular regions, internal mammary nodes, and any part of the axillary bed at risk
Tumor did not shrink enough to be removed with surgery	• Consider more systemic chemotherapy and/or preoperative radiation		• If tumor shrunk and surgery is possible, follow row above • If tumor did not shrink, treatment will be based on your doctor's recommendations

---

medical oncologist why one treatment might be preferred over another for your type of cancer.

For a list of adjuvant systemic therapy options based on preoperative treatment response, see Guide 19.

Guide 19
Adjuvant systemic therapy based on preoperative treatment response

ER+ and/or PR+ (hormone positive) with HER2-	• ypT0N0 or complete response • ypT1 to T4, N0 or residual disease • ypN1 (or more) or node positive	➡ • Endocrine therapy (see Guide 20)
ER- and/or PR- (hormone negative) with HER2+	• ypT0N0 or complete response	➡ • Complete up to one year of HER2-targeted therapy with trastuzumab alone or with pertuzumab (see Guide 21)
	• ypT1 to T4, N0 or residual disease • ypN1 (or more) or node positive	➡ • Ado-trastuzumab emtansine alone. If ado-trastuzumab emtansine discontinued for toxicity, then trastuzumab alone or with pertuzumab to complete one year of therapy.
ER+ and/or PR+ (hormone positive) with HER2+	• ypT0N0 or complete response	➡ • Endocrine therapy (see Guide 20) and complete up to one year of HER2-targeted therapy with trastuzumab alone or with pertuzumab (see Guide 21)
	• ypT1 to T4, N0 or residual disease • ypN1 (or more) or node positive	➡ • Ado-trastuzumab emtansine alone. If ado-trastuzumab emtansine discontinued for toxicity, then trastuzumab alone or with pertuzumab to complete one year of therapy. • Add endrocrine therapy (see Guide 20)
ER- and/or PR- with HER2- (TNBC)	• ypT0N0 or complete response	➡ • See follow-up care in Guide 23
	• ypT1 to T4, N0 or residual disease • ypN1 (or more) or node positive	➡ • Consider capecitabine

---

Hormone positive with HER2-

ER+ and/or PR+ is called hormone positive.
It is treated with adjuvant endocrine therapy
as found in Guide 20. When chemotherapy is
used, it is given before endocrine therapy.

Guide 20
Adjuvant endocrine therapy

Premenopause at diagnosis	• Tamoxifen alone for 5 years • Tamoxifen for 5 years with ovarian suppression or ablation	• After 5 years, if in postmenopause, then an aromatase inhibitor for 5 years or consider tamoxifen for another 5 years (for a total of 10 years on tamoxifen) • After 5 years, if still in premenopause, then consider tamoxifen for another 5 years (for a total of 10 years on tamoxifen) or stop endocrine therapy

• Aromatase inhibitor for 5 years with ovarian suppression or ablation

---

Postmenopause at diagnosis

• Aromatase inhibitor for 5 years, then consider aromatase inhibitor for 3 to 5 more years
• Aromatase inhibitor for 2 to 3 years, then tamoxifen to complete 5 years total of endocrine therapy
• Tamoxifen for 2 to 3 years, then an aromatase inhibitor to complete 5 years of endocrine therapy
• Tamoxifen for 2 to 3 years, then up to 5 years of an aromatase inhibitor

---

• Tamoxifen for 4.5 to 6 years, then an aromatase inhibitor for 5 years or consider tamoxifen for another 5 years (for a total of 10 years on tamoxifen)

• For those who can't have aromatase inhibitors or who don't want aromatase inhibitors, take tamoxifen for 5 years or consider tamoxifen for up to 10 years

---

Hormone negative with HER2+

ER- and/or PR- is called hormone negative. Since this cancer is HER2+, it is treated with targeted therapy.

- ➣ If no disease remains after preoperative therapy, then you will have up to one year of HER2-targeted therapy with trastuzumab alone or with pertuzumab

➣ If disease remains in the breast or there is cancer in the lymph nodes (node positive), then you will have ado-trastuzumab emtansine. If ado-trastuzumab emtansine is discontinued for toxicity, then you will receive trastuzumab alone or with pertuzumab to complete one year of therapy.

For HER2-targeted therapies, see Guide 21.

Guide 21
Systemic therapy for HER2+

Preferred options	• Doxorubicin and cyclophosphamide followed by paclitaxel with trastuzumab • Doxorubicin and cyclophosphamide followed by paclitaxel with trastuzumab and pertuzumab • Paclitaxel with trastuzumab • Docetaxel, carboplatin, and trastuzumab (TCH) • Docetaxel, carboplatin, trastuzumab, and pertuzumab (TCHP) • If no residual disease after preoperative therapy or no preoperative therapy: Complete up to one year of HER2-targeted therapy with trastuzumab alone or with pertuzumab • If residual disease after preoperative therapy: Ado-trastuzumab emtansine alone. If ado-trastuzumab emtansine discontinued for toxicity, then trastuzumab alone or with pertuzumab to complete one year of therapy.
Useful in some cases	• Docetaxel with cyclophosphamide and trastuzumab
Other recommended	• Doxorubicin with cyclophosphamide followed by docetaxel with trastuzumab • Doxorubicin with cyclophosphamide followed by docetaxel with trastuzumab and pertuzumab

Hormone positive with HER2+

Hormone positive with HER2+ is also called triple-positive breast cancer. Receptors for HER2, estrogen, and/or progesterone are found. It is treated with HER2-targeted therapy (see Guide 21) and endocrine therapy (see Guide 20).

> If no disease remains after preoperative therapy, then you will have endocrine therapy and up to one year of HER2-targeted therapy with trastuzumab alone or with pertuzumab.

> If disease remains or there is cancer in the lymph nodes (node positive), then you will have ado-trastuzumab emtansine. If ado-trastuzumab emtansine was discontinued for toxicity, then trastuzumab alone or with

pertuzumab will be given to complete one year of therapy. Endocrine therapy might be added.

Triple-negative breast cancer

In triple-negative breast cancer (TNBC), receptors for estrogen, progesterone, and HER2 are not found. This means the tumor has tested negative for HER2, estrogen hormone receptors, and progesterone receptors. It is written as ER- and/or PR- with HER2-. Systemic therapy options for HER- can be found in Guide 22.

This cancer does not respond to endocrine therapy or HER2-targeted therapy. If cancer remains, consider capecitabine. If no cancer remains, then see follow-up care in Guide 23.

Guide 22 Systemic therapy for HER2-	
Preferred options	• Doxorubicin and cyclophosphamide followed by paclitaxel • Docetaxel and cyclophosphamide (TC) • If triple-negative breast cancer (TNBC) and residual disease after preoperative chemotherapy (taxane, alkylating, or anthracycline), then use capecitabine
Useful in some cases	• Doxorubicin with cyclophosphamide • Cyclophosphamide, methotrexate, and fluorouracil (CMF) • Doxorubicin with cyclophosphamide followed by paclitaxel
Other recommended	• Doxorubicin and cyclophosphamide followed by docetaxel • Epirubicin and cyclophosphamide (EC) • Docetaxel, doxorubicin, and cyclophosphamide (TAC) • Select patients with TNBC in the preoperative setting only: paclitaxel with carboplatin or docetaxel with carboplatin

Follow-up care

After treatment, you will enter follow-up care. During this time, your health will be monitored for side effects of treatment and the return of cancer. This is part of your survivorship care plan.

It is important to keep follow-up visits and tests. Tell your doctor about any symptoms such as headaches or bone pain. Continue to take all medicine such as endocrine therapy exactly as prescribed and not miss or skip doses. You should receive a personalized survivorship care plan. It will provide a summary of possible long-term effects of treatment and list follow-up tests. Find out how your primary care provider will coordinate with specialists for your follow-up care.

Follow-up care can be found in Guide 23.

Guide 23
Follow-up care

Medical history and physical exam 1 to 4 times per year as needed for 5 years, then every year

Periodic screening for changes in family history

Genetic testing and referral to genetic counseling as needed

Monitor for lymphedema and refer for lymphedema management as needed

Mammogram every 12 months (not needed on reconstructed breast)

If signs and symptoms of metastases, then blood and imaging tests

If on endocrine therapy, continue to take endocrine therapy. Do not miss or skip doses.

Those with uterus and who are on tamoxifen should have a gynecology exam every 12 months

Those on an aromatase inhibitor or who later have ovarian failure should have bone density tests

Maintain an ideal weight, be active, eat a healthy diet, exercise, limit alcohol, and quit smoking

Review

> In stage 3 breast cancer, the cancer can be large and in the lymph nodes, the lymph nodes can be fixed (or not moveable), or the cancer can involve the skin or chest wall. It is not metastatic.

> Treatment before surgery is called preoperative therapy. It can be systemic therapy or radiation therapy. The goal of treatment is to shrink the tumor before surgery.

> Systemic therapy after surgery is called adjuvant therapy. Adjuvant therapy is based on how the tumor responded to preoperative treatment.

> All treatment is based on if the tumor has receptors for HER2, estrogen, and/or progesterone.

> In hormone-positive breast cancer, tests find hormone receptors for estrogen and/or progesterone on the tumor.

> Hormone-positive breast cancer is treated with endocrine therapy.

> HER2-positive (HER2+) breast cancer is treated with HER2-targeted therapy.

> It is important to keep follow-up visits and tests. Continue to take all medicine as prescribed.

7
Recurrence

72 Overview

72 Tests

73 Treatment

74 Review

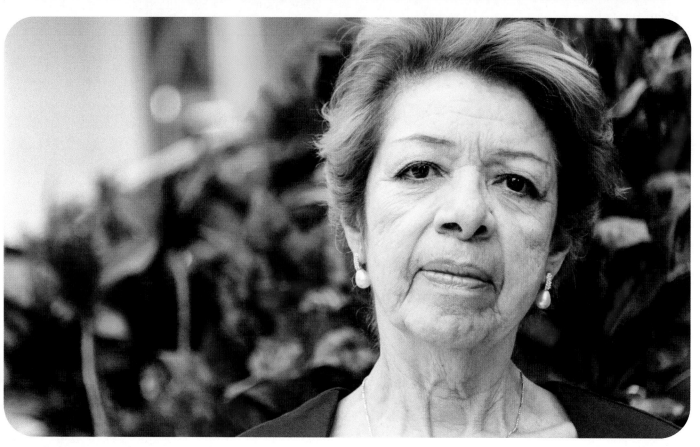

When cancer returns, it is called a recurrence. Treatment is based on the types of treatment you had before.

Overview

Breast cancer can return in 3 places:

> It can return to the breast that had cancer before. This is called a local recurrence.

> It can return to axillary lymph nodes or lymph nodes in or near the breast. This is called a regional occurrence.

> It can return in distant parts of the body. This is called metastatic breast cancer.

This chapter presents treatment options for local and regional recurrence.

When breast cancer has spread to distant parts of the body, it is called metastatic breast cancer. For more information, read the *NCCN Guidelines for Patients®: Breast Cancer – Metastatic* available at nccn.org/ patientguidelines.

Tests

You will have tests to decide which treatment options are right for you. This is called restaging. A biopsy is needed to confirm cancer. Tests such as a brain or spine MRI might be done based on your symptoms. Tests for recurrence can be found in Guide 24.

Guide 24
Testing for recurrence

Medical history and physical exam

Discuss goals of therapy and engage in shared decision-making

CBC and comprehensive metabolic panel (including liver function tests and alkaline phosphatase)

Chest CT with contrast (for diagnosis)

CT with contrast of abdomen with or without pelvis or MRI with contrast

Brain MRI with contrast if central nervous system (CNS) symptoms

Spine MRI with contrast if back pain or symptoms of spinal cord compression

Bone scan or sodium fluoride PET/CT, if needed

FDG PET/CT, if needed

X-rays if bone pain and if bones look abnormal on bone scan

First recurrence of disease should be biopsied

Determine tumor ER/PR and HER2 status on area of metastasis

Biomarker testing to identify those that would benefit from targeted therapy

Genetic counseling if at risk for hereditary breast cancer

Treatment

Treatment is based on where the cancer has returned and what type of treatment you had before. Surgery followed by radiation therapy (RT) and systemic therapy are possible. For treatment options, see Guide 25.

Some of the systemic therapy options have been described in this book. More information on recurrence can be found in *NCCN Guidelines for Patients®: Breast Cancer – Metastatic* available at nccn.org/patientguidelines.

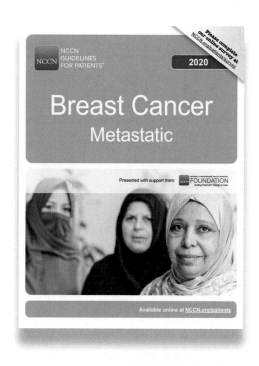

Guide 25	
Treatment for local and regional recurrence	
Local only	If first treatment lumpectomy with RT, then total mastectomy with axillary lymph node staging if level I and II axillary dissection not done before
	If first treatment mastectomy with level I and II axillary dissection and prior RT, then surgical resection if possible
	If first treatment mastectomy and no prior RT, then surgical resection if possible with RT
Regional only or Both local and regional recurrence	For axillary recurrence, surgical resection if possible with RT if possible
	For supraclavicular recurrence, RT if possible
	For internal mammary node recurrence, RT if possible

Local only

Treatment for a local recurrence is based on if your first treatment was a mastectomy or lumpectomy with or without radiation therapy (RT). More surgery might be an option. However, if you had RT before, then it may not be possible to have it again in the same area.

Regional only

Treatment for a regional-only recurrence is RT when possible. If the regional recurrence is in or near the armpit (axilla), then surgery to remove the tumor might be an option before RT.

Both local and regional

Cancer that is both local and regional might be referred to as a locoregional recurrence. Treatment for a locoregional recurrence is surgery followed by radiation (if it is possible to give more radiation). Some people receive preoperative therapy if surgery is not possible. Chemotherapy before radiation might be given for supraclavicular and internal mammary node recurrence.

Review

> When cancer returns, it is called a recurrence.

> Cancer that returns to the breast that had cancer before is called a local recurrence.

> Cancer that returns to axillary lymph nodes or lymph nodes in or near the breast is called a regional recurrence.

> Cancer that returns in distant parts of the body is called metastatic breast cancer.

> Treatment is based on where the cancer has returned and what type of treatment you had before.

> Surgery followed by radiation therapy and systemic therapy are possible.

> More information on recurrence can be found in *NCCN Guidelines for Patients®: Breast Cancer – Metastatic* available at nccn.org/patientguidelines.

8
Inflammatory breast cancer

76   Overview

77   Tests

78   Treatment

84   Review

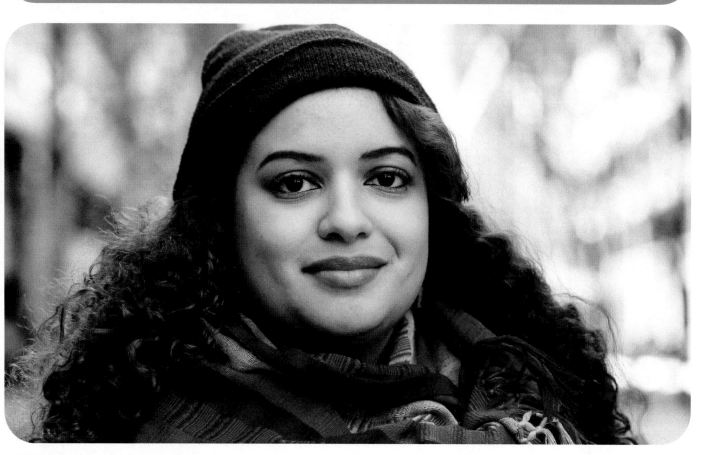

In inflammatory breast cancer (IBC), cancer cells block lymph vessels in the skin of the breast. This causes the breast to look red and swollen and feel warm to the touch. Treatment is systemic therapy to shrink the tumor, followed by surgery to remove the tumor, and then radiation. Together, you and your doctor will choose a treatment plan that is best for you.

Overview

Most inflammatory breast cancers (IBCs) are invasive ductal carcinomas. This means that cancer started in the cells that line the milk ducts and has spread into surrounding tissue. At diagnosis, IBC is stage 3 or 4 disease. In stage 3, cancer may be in nearby lymph nodes. In stage 4, cancer is in nearby lymph nodes and has spread to other parts of the body (metastasized).

Since IBC spreads quickly, treatment starts with systemic therapy to stop the spread of cancer. Radiation might follow systemic therapy. If the cancer responds to treatment, then surgery to remove the breast (mastectomy) will be done. If radiation is used after a mastectomy, delayed reconstruction is an option. Radiation can slow the healing process.

Like other breast cancers, IBC can happen in men.

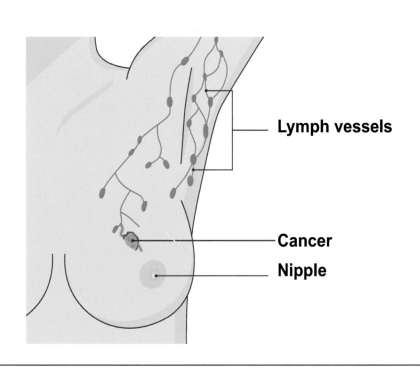

Lymph vessels

Lymph is a clear fluid. It drains from breast tissue into lymph vessels where it travels to lymph nodes. In inflammatory breast cancer, cancer cells block lymph vessels in the skin of the breast.

Lymph vessels

Cancer

Nipple

Tests

IBC can be difficult to diagnose. Often, there is no lump that can be felt during a breast exam or seen on a mammogram. Since there is swelling and redness of the breast, IBC can look like an infection and therefore be difficult to diagnose.

You will have blood tests, imaging tests, and a biopsy to stage the cancer. The biopsy sample will be tested for hormone receptors and HER2 receptors. Treatment will be based on these findings.

Imaging and staging tests may include the following:

> A mammogram and an ultrasound of the breast and regional (nearby) lymph nodes

> A CT scan or a PET/CT scan and a bone scan to see if the cancer has spread to other parts of the body

Tests for IBC can be found in Guide 26.

Guide 26	
Testing for inflammatory breast cancer (IBC)	
Needed	• Medical history and physical exam by multidisciplinary team • CBC and comprehensive metabolic panel (including liver function tests and alkaline phosphatase) • Determine tumor ER/PR and HER2 status • Diagnostic mammogram • Fertility counseling if in premenopause • Bone scan or sodium fluoride PET/CT • CT with contrast of chest/abdomen/pelvis • Genetic counseling if at risk for hereditary breast cancer
Other	• Ultrasound of breast • Breast MRI • FDG PET/CT

Treatment

Treatment for IBC starts with preoperative systemic therapy. Preoperative therapy is treatment given before surgery. It is based on if the tumor is HER2+ or HER2-.

For HER2- cancer, the preferred treatment is an anthracycline with a taxane. These are types of chemotherapy. Anthracyclines include doxorubicin and epirubicin. Docetaxel, paclitaxel, and albumin-bound paclitaxel are taxanes.

IBCs often produce greater than normal amounts of HER2. If the tumor is HER2+, then HER2-targeted therapy should be given as preoperative systemic therapy.

Preoperative systemic therapy options for HER2+ can be found in Guide 27.

Guide 27
Systemic therapy for HER2+

Preferred options	• Doxorubicin and cyclophosphamide followed by paclitaxel with trastuzumab • Doxorubicin and cyclophosphamide followed by paclitaxel with trastuzumab and pertuzumab • Paclitaxel with trastuzumab • Docetaxel, carboplatin, and trastuzumab (TCH) • Docetaxel, carboplatin, trastuzumab, and pertuzumab (TCHP) • If no residual disease after preoperative therapy or no preoperative therapy: Complete up to one year of HER2-targeted therapy with trastuzumab alone or with pertuzumab • If residual disease after preoperative therapy: Ado-trastuzumab emtansine alone. If ado-trastuzumab emtansine discontinued for toxicity, then trastuzumab alone or with pertuzumab to complete one year of therapy.
Useful in some cases	• Docetaxel with cyclophosphamide and trastuzumab
Other recommended	• Doxorubicin with cyclophosphamide followed by docetaxel with trastuzumab • Doxorubicin with cyclophosphamide followed by docetaxel with trastuzumab and pertuzumab

Preoperative systemic therapy options for
HER2- can be found in Guide 28.

Guide 28 Systemic therapy for HER2-	
Preferred options	• Doxorubicin and cyclophosphamide followed by paclitaxel • Docetaxel and cyclophosphamide (TC) • If triple-negative breast cancer (TNBC) and residual disease after preoperative chemotherapy (taxane, alkylating, or anthracycline), then use capecitabine
Useful in some cases	• Doxorubicin with cyclophosphamide • Cyclophosphamide, methotrexate, and fluorouracil (CMF) • Doxorubicin with cyclophosphamide followed by paclitaxel
Other recommended	• Doxorubicin and cyclophosphamide followed by docetaxel • Epirubicin and cyclophosphamide (EC) • Docetaxel, doxorubicin, and cyclophosphamide (TAC) • Select patients with TNBC in the preoperative setting only: paclitaxel with carboplatin or docetaxel with carboplatin

Treatment response

The next treatment is based on how the tumor responded to preoperative systemic therapy. It is called preoperative (before surgery) treatment because the goal is surgery, when possible. Systemic treatment after surgery is called adjuvant therapy.

A physical exam and imaging tests should be done to assess how the cancer responded to preoperative systemic therapy. Treatment will be based on if the tumor shrunk and surgery is possible or if the tumor did not shrink enough to be removed with surgery. See Guide 29.

Surgery is an option

If the tumor shrunk enough so surgery is possible, then a total mastectomy with level I and II axillary lymph node dissection is the recommended option. You may choose a delayed breast reconstruction as part of the mastectomy. Radiation therapy (RT) is part of this treatment.

After the mastectomy and RT, you will finish chemotherapy if you didn't complete the course before surgery. If the tumor is ER+ and/or PR+, then you will have endocrine therapy. Endocrine therapy is used to treat

---

Guide 29
IBC treatment options based on preoperative treatment response

Tumor shrunk and surgery is possible	• Total mastectomy with level I and II axillary dissection with radiation therapy to chest wall, infraclavicular region, supraclavicular area, internal mammary nodes, and any part of the axillary bed at risk • Breast reconstruction (delayed) is optional	• Complete planned chemotherapy regimen course if not completed preoperatively plus endocrine treatment if ER+ and/or PR+ (sequential chemotherapy followed by endocrine therapy) • If HER2+, complete up to one year of HER2-targeted therapy. This may be given with RT and with endocrine therapy
Tumor did not shrink enough to be removed with surgery	• Consider more systemic chemotherapy (see Guide 31 and Guide 32) and/or preoperative radiation	• If tumor shrunk and surgery is possible, follow section above • If tumor did not shrink, treatment will be based on your doctor's recommendations

---

tumors that are estrogen-positive (ER+) and/or progesterone-positive (PR+).

If the tumor is HER2+, then you will have up to one year of HER2-targeted therapy. This may be given with RT and endocrine therapy.

For a list of systemic therapies that target HER2+, see Guide 27.

For a list of adjuvant endocrine therapies, see Guide 30.

Guide 30
Adjuvant endocrine therapy

Premenopause at diagnosis	• Tamoxifen alone for 5 years • Tamoxifen for 5 years with ovarian suppression or ablation →	• After 5 years, if in postmenopause, then an aromatase inhibitor for 5 years or consider tamoxifen for another 5 years (for a total of 10 years on tamoxifen) • After 5 years, if still in premenopause, then consider tamoxifen for another 5 years (for a total of 10 years on tamoxifen) or stop endocrine therapy
	• Aromatase inhibitor for 5 years with ovarian suppression or ablation	
Postmenopause at diagnosis	• Aromatase inhibitor for 5 years, then consider aromatase inhibitor for 3 to 5 more years • Aromatase inhibitor for 2 to 3 years, then tamoxifen to complete 5 years total of endocrine therapy • Tamoxifen for 2 to 3 years, then an aromatase inhibitor to complete 5 years of endocrine therapy • Tamoxifen for 2 to 3 years, then up to 5 years of an aromatase inhibitor	
	• Tamoxifen for 4.5 to 6 years, then an aromatase inhibitor for 5 years or consider tamoxifen for another 5 years (for a total of 10 years on tamoxifen)	
	• For those who can't have aromatase inhibitors or who don't want aromatase inhibitors, take tamoxifen for 5 years or consider tamoxifen for up to 10 years	

Surgery is not an option

Surgery is not always possible. Even though surgery might not be an option, systemic therapy will continue. If the cancer is not responding to systemic therapy, then radiation may be considered to try to make the cancer resectable. The goal of treatment is to reduce the amount of cancer. Talk with your doctor about your goals of treatment and your treatment preferences. Your wishes are always important.

For a list of systemic therapies that target HER2+, see Guide 31.

Guide 31	
Systemic therapy for HER+	
Preferred options	• Pertuzumab, trastuzumab, and docetaxel • Pertuzumab, trastuzumab, and paclitaxel
Other recommended	• Ado-trastuzumab emtansine (T-DM1) • Fam-trastuzumab deruxtecan-nxki • Trastuzumab and paclitaxel with or without carboplatin • Trastuzumab and docetaxel • Trastuzumab and vinorelbine • Trastuzumab and capecitabine • Lapatinib and capecitabine • Trastuzumab and lapatinib (without cytotoxic therapy) • Trastuzumab with other agents • Neratinib and capecitabine • For *BRCA1* or *BRCA2* mutations, olaparib or talazoparib • For *NTRK* fusion, larotrectinib or entrectinib • For MSI-H/dMMR, pembrolizumab

For a list of systemic therapies for HER2-, see Guide 32.

Guide 32
Systemic therapy for HER-

Preferred options	• Anthracyclines (doxorubicin or liposomal doxorubicin) • Taxanes such as paclitaxel • Antimetabolites (capecitabine or gemcitabine) • Microtubule inhibitors (vinorelbine or eribulin) • For *BRCA1* or *BRCA2* mutations, olararib or talazoparib • For *BRCA1* or *BRCA2* mutations, platinum (carboplatin or cisplatin) • For *NTRK* fusion, larotrectinib or entrectinib • For MSI-H/dMMR, pembrolizumab • For PD-L1 expression of more than 1%, atezolizumab with albumin-bound paclitaxel
Other recommended	• Cyclophosphamide • Docetaxel • Albumin-bound paclitaxel • Epirubicin • Ixabepilone
Used in some cases	• AC (doxorubicin with cyclophosphamide) • EC (epirubicin with cyclophosphamide) • CMF (cyclophosphamide with methotrexate and fluorouracil) • Docetaxel with capecitabine • GT (gemcitabine with paclitaxel) • Gemcitabine with carboplatin • Paclitaxel with bevacizumab • Carboplatin with paclitaxel or albumin-bound paclitaxel

Review

> In inflammatory breast cancer (IBC), cancer cells block lymph vessels in the skin of the breast. This causes the breast to look red and swollen and feel warm to the touch.

> IBC is treated with systemic therapy to shrink the tumor, followed by surgery to remove the tumor, and then radiation. Surgery is not always possible. Even though surgery might not be an option, systemic therapy will continue.

> Treatment is based on blood tests, imaging tests, and a biopsy to stage the cancer. The biopsy sample will be tested for hormone receptors and HER2 receptors.

> IBCs often produce greater than normal amounts of HER2. If the tumor is HER2+, then HER2-targeted therapy may be given as preoperative systemic therapy.

> Endocrine therapy is used to treat tumors that are estrogen-positive (ER+) and/or progesterone-positive (PR+).

> Systemic therapy given after surgery is called adjuvant therapy. Adjuvant systemic therapy may be given after surgery to reduce the chance of cancer recurrence.

9
Making treatment decisions

86   It's your choice

86   Questions to ask your doctors

92   Websites

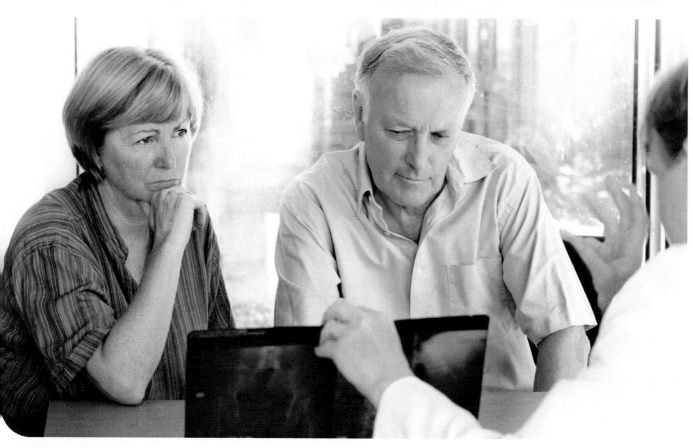

It's important to be comfortable with the cancer treatment you choose. This choice starts with having an open and honest conversation with your doctor.

It's your choice

In shared decision-making, you and your doctors share information, discuss the options, and agree on a treatment plan. It starts with an open and honest conversation between you and your doctor.

Treatment decisions are very personal. What is important to you may not be important to someone else.

Some things that may play a role in your decision-making:

- What you want and how that might differ from what others want

- Your religious and spiritual beliefs

- Your feelings about certain treatments like surgery or chemotherapy

- Your feelings about pain or side effects such as nausea and vomiting

- Cost of treatment, travel to treatment centers, and time away from work

- Quality of life and length of life

- How active you are and the activities that are important to you

Think about what you want from treatment. Discuss openly the risks and benefits of specific treatments and procedures. Weigh options and share concerns with your doctor. If you take the time to build a relationship with your doctor, it will help you feel supported when considering options and making treatment decisions.

Second opinion

It is normal to want to start treatment as soon as possible. While cancer can't be ignored, there is time to have another doctor review your test results and suggest a treatment plan. This is called getting a second opinion, and it's a normal part of cancer care. Even doctors get second opinions!

Things you can do to prepare:

- Check with your insurance company about its rules on second opinions. There may be out-of-pocket costs to see doctors who are not part of your insurance plan.

- Make plans to have copies of all your records sent to the doctor you will see for your second opinion.

Support groups

Many people diagnosed with cancer find support groups to be helpful. Support groups often include people at different stages of treatment. Some people may be newly diagnosed, while others may be finished with treatment. If your hospital or community doesn't have support groups for people with cancer, check out the websites listed in this book.

Questions to ask your doctors

Possible questions to ask your doctors are listed on the following pages. Feel free to use these questions or come up with your own. Be clear about your goals for treatment and find out what to expect from treatment.

Questions to ask about diagnosis and prognosis

1. Where did the cancer start? In what type of cell? Is this cancer common?

2. Is this a fast- or slow-growing cancer?

3. What stage is the breast cancer? What does this mean?

4. What tests do you recommend for me? Will I have any genetic tests?

5. What will you do to make me comfortable during testing?

6. What if I am pregnant or want to become pregnant?

7. Would you give me a copy of the pathology report and other test results?

8. How soon will I know the results and who will explain them to me?

9. Who will talk with me about the next steps? When?

10. What can I do before my next appointment?

Questions to ask about options

1. What will happen if I do nothing?

2. How do my age, overall health, and other factors affect my options?

3. What if I am pregnant? What if I'm planning to get pregnant in the near future?

4. Which option is proven to work best?

5. Does any option offer a cure or long-term cancer control? Are my chances any better for one option than another? Less time-consuming? Less expensive? What does my health insurance cover?

6. What are the possible complications and side effects?

7. Is surgery an option? Why or why not?

8. How do you know if treatment is working? How will I know if treatment is working?

9. What are my options if my treatment stops working?

10. What can be done to prevent or relieve the side effects of treatment?

11. Are there any life-threatening side effects of this treatment? How will I be monitored?

12. Can I stop treatment at any time? What will happen if I stop treatment?

13. Are there any clinical trials I should consider for my condition?

Questions to ask about treatment

1. What are my treatment choices? What are the benefits and risks?

2. Which treatment do you recommend and why?

3. How long do I have to decide?

4. Will I have to go to the hospital or elsewhere for treatment? How often? How long is each visit? Will I have to stay overnight in the hospital or make travel plans?

5. Do I have a choice of when to begin treatment? Can I choose the days and times of treatment? Should I bring someone with me?

6. How much will the treatment hurt? What will you do to make me comfortable?

7. How much will this treatment cost me? What does my insurance cover? Are there any programs to help me pay for treatment?

8. Will I miss work or school? Will I be able to drive?

9. What type of home care will I need? What kind of treatment will I need to do at home?

10. When will I be able to return to my normal activities?

11. Which treatment will give me the best quality of life? Which treatment will extend my life? By how long?

12. I would like a second opinion. Is there someone you can recommend? Who can help me gather all of my records for a second opinion?

Questions to ask about clinical trials

1. What clinical trials are available for my type and stage of breast cancer?

2. What are the treatments used in the clinical trial?

3. What does the treatment do?

4. Has the treatment been used before? Has it been used for other types of cancer?

5. What are the risks and benefits of this treatment?

6. What side effects should I expect? How will the side effects be controlled?

7. How long will I be on the clinical trial?

8. Will I be able to get other treatment if this doesn't work?

9. How will you know the treatment is working?

10. Will the clinical trial cost me anything? If so, how much?

11. How do I find out about clinical trials that I can participate in? Are there online sources that I can search?

Questions to ask about side effects

1. What are the side effects of treatment?

2. How long will these side effects last?

3. What side effects should I watch for?

4. When should I call the doctor about my side effects? Can I text?

5. What medicines can I take to prevent or relieve side effects?

6. What can I do to help with pain and other side effects?

7. Will you stop treatment or change treatment if I have side effects?

8. What can I do to prevent side effects? What will you do?

Websites

American Cancer Society
cancer.org/cancer/breast-cancer.html

Breast Cancer Alliance
breastcanceralliance.org

Breastcancer.org
breastcancer.org

Breast Cancer Trials
breastcancertrials.org

DiepCFoundation
diepcfoundation.org

FORCE: Facing Our Risk of Cancer Empowered
facingourrisk.org

Living Beyond Breast Cancer (LBBC)
lbbc.org

National Cancer Institute (NCI)
cancer.gov/types/breast

Sharsheret
sharsheret.org

Young Survival Coalition (YSC)
youngsurvival.org

Looking for help to quit smoking?

✓ Smokefree.gov
✓ BeTobaccoFree.gov

Words to know

adjuvant therapy
Treatment that is given to lower the chances of the cancer returning.

anti-estrogen
A cancer drug that stops estrogen from attaching to cells.

areola
A darker, round area of skin on the breast around the nipple.

aromatase inhibitor
A drug that lowers the level of estrogen in the body.

axillary lymph node (ALN)
A small disease-fighting structure that is near the armpit.

axillary lymph node dissection (ALND)
An operation that removes the disease-fighting structures (lymph nodes) near the armpit.

bilateral diagnostic mammogram
Pictures of the insides of both breasts that are made from a set of x-rays.

bilateral oophorectomy
An operation that removes both ovaries.

biopsy
A procedure that removes fluid or tissue samples to be tested for a disease.

bone mineral density
A test that measures the strength of bones.

bone scan
A test that makes pictures of bones to assess for health problems.

boost
An extra dose of radiation to a specific area of the body.

breast implant
A small bag filled with salt water, gel, or both that is used to remake breasts.

breast reconstruction
An operation that creates new breasts.

breast-conserving therapy
A cancer treatment that includes removing a breast lump and radiation therapy.

cancer stage
A rating of the outlook of a cancer based on its growth and spread.

carcinoma
A cancer of cells that line the inner or outer surfaces of the body.

chemotherapy
Cancer drugs that stop the cell life cycle so cells don't increase in number.

chest wall
The layer of muscle, bone, and fat that protects the vital organs.

clinical breast exam
Touching of a breast by a health expert to feel for diseases.

clinical stage
The rating of the extent of cancer before treatment is started.

clinical trial
A type of research that assesses health tests or treatments.

complete blood count (CBC)
A lab test that includes the number of blood cells.

computed tomography (CT)
A test that uses x-rays from many angles to make a picture of the insides of the body.

contrast
A substance put into your body to make clearer pictures during imaging tests.

core needle biopsy
A procedure that removes tissue samples with a hollow needle. Also called core biopsy.

deoxyribonucleic acid (DNA)
A chain of chemicals in cells that contains coded instructions for making and controlling cells. Also called the "blueprint of life."

diagnostic bilateral mammogram
Pictures of the insides of both breasts that are made from a set of x-rays.

duct
A tube-shaped structure through which milk travels to the nipple.

ductal carcinoma
A cancer derived from cells that line small tube-shaped vessels.

endocrine therapy
A cancer treatment that stops the making or action of estrogen. Also called hormone therapy.

estrogen
A hormone that causes female body traits.

fertility specialist
An expert who helps people to have babies.

fine-needle aspiration (FNA)
A procedure that removes tissue samples with a very thin needle.

gene
Coded instructions in cells for making new cells and controlling how cells behave.

genetic counseling
Expert guidance on the chance for a disease that is passed down in families.

hereditary breast cancer
Breast cancer that was likely caused by abnormal genes passed down from parent to child.

histology
The structure of cells, tissue, and organs as viewed under a microscope.

hormone
A chemical in the body that triggers a response from cells or organs.

hormone receptor-negative cancer (HR-)
Cancer cells that don't use hormones to grow.

hormone receptor-positive cancer (HR+)
Cancer cells that use hormones to grow.

human epidermal growth factor receptor 2 (HER2)
A protein on the edge of a cell that sends signals for the cell to grow.

imaging test
A test that makes pictures (images) of the insides of the body.

immune system
The body's natural defense against infection and disease.

immunohistochemistry (IHC)
A lab test of cancer cells to find specific cell traits involved in abnormal cell growth.

in situ hybridization (ISH)
A lab test of the number of a gene.

infraclavicular
The area right below the collarbone.

internal mammary
The area along the breastbone.

invasive breast cancer
The growth of breast cancer into the breast's supporting tissue (stroma).

lobular carcinoma
A breast cancer that started in cells that line the breast glands (lobules).

lobule
A gland in the breast that makes breast milk.

lumpectomy
An operation that removes a small breast cancer tumor.

luteinizing hormone-releasing hormone (LHRH)
A hormone in the brain that helps control the making of estrogen by the ovaries.

lymph
A clear fluid containing white blood cells.

lymph node
A small, bean-shaped, disease-fighting structure.

lymphedema
Swelling in the body due to a buildup of fluid called lymph.

magnetic resonance imaging (MRI)
A test that uses radio waves and powerful magnets to make pictures of the insides of the body.

mammogram
A picture of the insides of the breast that is made by an x-ray test.

mastectomy
An operation that removes the whole breast.

medical history
A report of all your health events and medications.

medical oncologist
A doctor who's an expert in cancer drugs.

menopause
The point in time when menstrual periods end.

mutation
An abnormal change.

neoadjuvant treatment
A treatment that is given before the main treatment to reduce the cancer. Also called preoperative treatment if given before an operation.

noninvasive breast cancer
Breast cancer that has not grown into tissue from which it can spread.

ovarian ablation
Methods used to stop the ovaries from making hormones.

ovarian suppression
A drug treatment that lowers the amount of hormones made by the ovaries.

partial breast irradiation
Treatment with radiation that is received at the site of the removed breast tumor.

pathologic stage
A rating of the extent of cancer based on tests given after treatment.

pathologist
A doctor who's an expert in testing cells and tissue to find disease.

pelvis
The body area between the hipbones.

physical exam
A study of the body by a health expert for signs of disease.

positron emission tomography (PET)
A test that uses radioactive material to see the shape and function of body parts.

postmenopausal
The state of having no more menstrual periods

premenopause
The state of having regular menstrual periods.

primary tumor
The first mass of cancer cells.

progesterone
A hormone in women that is involved in sexual development, periods, and pregnancy.

prognosis
The likely course and outcome of a disease based on tests.

radiation therapy (RT)
A treatment that uses high-energy rays.

recurrence
The return of cancer after a cancer-free period.

selective estrogen receptor modulator (SERM)
A drug that blocks the effect of estrogen inside of cells.

sentinel lymph node
The first lymph node to which cancer cells spread after leaving a tumor.

sentinel lymph node biopsy (SLNB)
An operation to remove the disease-fighting structures (lymph nodes) to which cancer first spreads. Also called sentinel lymph node dissection.

side effect
An unhealthy or unpleasant physical or emotional response to treatment.

skin-sparing mastectomy
An operation that removes all breast tissue but saves as much breast skin as possible.

supportive care
Health care that includes symptom relief but not cancer treatment. Also called palliative care.

supraclavicular
The area right above the collarbone.

surgical margin
The normal-looking tissue around a tumor that was removed during an operation.

systemic therapy
A type of treatment that works throughout the body.

total mastectomy
An operation that removes the entire breast but no chest muscles. Also called simple mastectomy.

triple-negative breast cancer (TNBC)
A breast cancer that does not use hormones or the HER2 protein to grow.

ultrasound
A test that uses sound waves to take pictures of the inside of the body.

volume displacement
A method to shift breast tissue during an operation to fill a gap.

whole breast radiation therapy (WBRT)
Treatment with radiation of the entire breast.

NCCN Contributors

This patient guide is based on the NCCN Clinical Practice Guidelines in Oncology (NCCN Guidelines®) for Breast Cancer. It was adapted, reviewed, and published with help from the following people:

Dorothy A. Shead, MS
Director, Patient Information Operations

Laura J. Hanisch, PsyD
Medical Writer/Patient Information Specialist

Erin Vidic, MA
Medical Writer

Rachael Clarke
Senior Medical Copyeditor

Tanya Fischer, MEd, MSLIS
Medical Writer

Kim Williams
Creative Services Manager

Susan Kidney
Design Specialist

The NCCN Clinical Practice Guidelines in Oncology (NCCN Guidelines®) for Breast Cancer, Version 3.2020 were developed by the following NCCN Panel Members:

William J. Gradishar, MD/Chair
Robert H. Lurie Comprehensive Cancer Center of Northwestern University

Benjamin O. Anderson, MD/Vice-Chair
Fred Hutchinson Cancer Research Center/Seattle Cancer Care Alliance

Jame Abraham, MD
Case Comprehensive Cancer Center/ University Hospitals Seidman Cancer Center and Cleveland Clinic Taussig Cancer Institute

*Rebecca Aft, MD, PhD
Siteman Cancer Center at Barnes-Jewish Hospital and Washington University School of Medicine

Doreen Agnese, MD
The Ohio State University Comprehensive Cancer Center - James Cancer Hospital and Solove Research Institute

Kimberly H. Allison, MD
Stanford Cancer Institute

*Sarah L. Blair, MD
UC San Diego Moores Cancer Center

Harold J. Burstein, MD, PhD
Dana-Farber/Brigham and Women's Cancer Center

Chau Dang, MD
Memorial Sloan Kettering Cancer Center

Anthony D. Elias, MD
University of Colorado Cancer Center

Sharon H. Giordano, MD, MPH
The University of Texas MD Anderson Cancer Center

Matthew Goetz, MD
Mayo Clinic Cancer Center

Lori J. Goldstein, MD
Fox Chase Cancer Center

Steven J. Isakoff, MD, PhD
Massachusetts General Hospital Cancer Center

Jairam Krishnamurthy, MD
Fred & Pamela Buffet Cancer Center

*Janice Lyons, MD
Case Comprehensive Cancer Center/ University Hospitals Seidman Cancer Center and Cleveland Clinic Taussig Cancer Institute

P. Kelly Marcom, MD
Duke Cancer Institute

Jennifer Matro, MD
Abramson Cancer Center at the University of Pennsylvania

Ingrid A. Mayer, MD
Vanderbilt-Ingram Cancer Center

Meena S. Moran, MD
Yale Cancer Center/Smilow Cancer Hospital

Joanne Mortimer, MD
City of Hope National Medical Center

Ruth M. O'Regan, MD
University of Wisconsin Carbone Cancer Center

Sameer A. Patel, MD
Fox Chase Cancer Center

Lori J. Pierce, MD
University of Michigan Rogel Cancer Center

Hope S. Rugo, MD
UCSF Helen Diller Family Comprehensive Cancer Center

Amy Sitapati, MD
UC San Diego Moores Cancer Center

Karen Lisa Smith, MD, MPH
The Sidney Kimmel Comprehensive Cancer Center at Johns Hopkins

*Mary Lou Smith, JD, MBA
Patient Advocate Research Advocacy Network

Hatem Soliman, MD
Moffitt Cancer Center

Erica M. Stringer-Reasor, MD
O'Neal Comprehensive Cancer Center at UAB

Melinda L. Telli, MD
Stanford Cancer Institute

John H. Ward, MD
Huntsman Cancer Institute at the University of Utah

Jessica S. Young, MD
Roswell Park Comprehensive Cancer Center

NCCN Staff

Rashmi Kumar, PhD
Director, Clinical Information Operations

Jennifer Burns, BS
Manager, Guidelines Support

* Reviewed this patient guide.
For disclosures, visit NCCN.org/about/disclosure.aspx.

NCCN Guidelines for Patients®:
Invasive Breast Cancer, 2020

NCCN Cancer Centers

Abramson Cancer Center
at the University of Pennsylvania
Philadelphia, Pennsylvania
800.789.7366 • pennmedicine.org/cancer

Fred & Pamela Buffett Cancer Center
Omaha, Nebraska
800.999.5465 • nebraskamed.com/cancer

Case Comprehensive Cancer Center/
University Hospitals Seidman Cancer
Center and Cleveland Clinic Taussig
Cancer Institute
Cleveland, Ohio
800.641.2422 • UH Seidman Cancer Center
uhhospitals.org/services/cancer-services
866.223.8100 • CC Taussig Cancer Institute
my.clevelandclinic.org/departments/cancer
216.844.8797 • Case CCC
case.edu/cancer

City of Hope National Medical Center
Los Angeles, California
800.826.4673 • cityofhope.org

Dana-Farber/Brigham and
Women's Cancer Center
Massachusetts General Hospital
Cancer Center
Boston, Massachusetts
877.332.4294
dfbwcc.org
massgeneral.org/cancer

Duke Cancer Institute
Durham, North Carolina
888.275.3853 • dukecancerinstitute.org

Fox Chase Cancer Center
Philadelphia, Pennsylvania
888.369.2427 • foxchase.org

Huntsman Cancer Institute
at the University of Utah
Salt Lake City, Utah
877.585.0303
huntsmancancer.org

Fred Hutchinson Cancer
Research Center/Seattle
Cancer Care Alliance
Seattle, Washington
206.288.7222 • seattlecca.org
206.667.5000 • fredhutch.org

The Sidney Kimmel Comprehensive
Cancer Center at Johns Hopkins
Baltimore, Maryland
410.955.8964
hopkinskimmelcancercenter.org

Robert H. Lurie Comprehensive
Cancer Center of Northwestern
University
Chicago, Illinois
866.587.4322 • cancer.northwestern.edu

Mayo Clinic Cancer Center
Phoenix/Scottsdale, Arizona
Jacksonville, Florida
Rochester, Minnesota
800.446.2279 • Arizona
904.953.0853 • Florida
507.538.3270 • Minnesota
mayoclinic.org/departments-centers/mayo-clinic-cancer-center

Memorial Sloan Kettering
Cancer Center
New York, New York
800.525.2225 • mskcc.org

Moffitt Cancer Center
Tampa, Florida
800.456.3434 • moffitt.org

The Ohio State University
Comprehensive Cancer Center -
James Cancer Hospital and
Solove Research Institute
Columbus, Ohio
800.293.5066 • cancer.osu.edu

O'Neal Comprehensive
Cancer Center at UAB
Birmingham, Alabama
800.822.0933 • uab.edu/onealcancercenter

Roswell Park Comprehensive
Cancer Center
Buffalo, New York
877.275.7724 • roswellpark.org

Siteman Cancer Center at Barnes-
Jewish Hospital and Washington
University School of Medicine
St. Louis, Missouri
800.600.3606 • siteman.wustl.edu

St. Jude Children's Research Hospital
The University of Tennessee
Health Science Center
Memphis, Tennessee
888.226.4343 • stjude.org
901.683.0055 • westclinic.com

Stanford Cancer Institute
Stanford, California
877.668.7535 • cancer.stanford.edu

UC San Diego Moores Cancer Center
La Jolla, California
858.657.7000 • cancer.ucsd.edu

UCLA Jonsson
Comprehensive Cancer Center
Los Angeles, California
310.825.5268 • cancer.ucla.edu

UCSF Helen Diller Family
Comprehensive Cancer Center
San Francisco, California
800.689.8273 • cancer.ucsf.edu

University of Colorado Cancer Center
Aurora, Colorado
720.848.0300 • coloradocancercenter.org

University of Michigan
Rogel Cancer Center
Ann Arbor, Michigan
800.865.1125 • rogelcancercenter.org

The University of Texas
MD Anderson Cancer Center
Houston, Texas
800.392.1611 • mdanderson.org

University of Wisconsin
Carbone Cancer Center
Madison, Wisconsin
608.265.1700 • uwhealth.org/cancer

UT Southwestern Simmons
Comprehensive Cancer Center
Dallas, Texas
214.648.3111 • utswmed.org/cancer

Vanderbilt-Ingram Cancer Center
Nashville, Tennessee
800.811.8480 • vicc.org

Yale Cancer Center/
Smilow Cancer Hospital
New Haven, Connecticut
855.4.SMILOW • yalecancercenter.org

axillary lymph node (ALN) 7, 10, 21

axillary lymph node dissection (ALND) 21

biopsy 19–21

birth control 16, 34

blood tests 17

bone scan 18

bone-targeted therapy 35

breast-conserving therapy (see lumpectomy)

breast reconstruction 42–43

cancer stages 9–12

chemotherapy 34

clinical stage 9-10

clinical trial 37

computed tomography (CT) 17

distress 25

endocrine therapy 31–32

family history 15

fertility 16

genetic counseling 24–25

hereditary breast cancer 24–25

histology 50, 58

hormone receptor 22–23

human epidermal growth factor receptor 2 (HER2) 23, 33

imaging tests 17–19

immunohistochemistry (IHC) 22

inoperable 61, 64

lumpectomy 29

lymphedema 38

magnetic resonance imaging (MRI) 18

mammogram 17

mastectomy 30

menopause 32

metastatic breast cancer 8–12, 72

medical history 15

micrometastasis 12, 48

mutations 23–25

operable 61–62

pathologic stage 9, 64

physical exam 15

positron emission tomography (PET) 18–19

postmenopause 32

pregnancy 16–17, 34

premenopause 32

radiation therapy (RT) 30

recurrence 24

sentinel lymph node biopsy (SLNB) 20

supportive care 38

triple-negative breast cancer (TNBC) 54, 60, 68

tumor tests 24

ultrasound 18

Made in the USA
Coppell, TX
04 November 2020

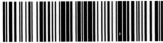